Ageless Athletic Assassin

How Martial Arts Saved Me from Bullying, Racism, Obesity, and Mediocrity

FRANCIS HUYNH

WARNING

Reading this book may significantly improve your health.
Side Effects: Motivation to become sexy, strong, and smart.

The information of this book is not intended to take the place of medical advice from your healthcare provider. Readers are strongly advised to consult with their doctor or other healthcare provider before altering or undertaking any exercise or nutritional program or before taking any medication or supplement referred to in this book. Any application of the recommendations set forth in the following pages is at the reader's discretion and sole risk.

DEDICATION

I dedicate this book to my wife, parents, and family who've supported me in forgoing lucrative post-MBA corporate careers and delaying having kids with my married wife in 2016 to pursue my calling of helping the 2 billion overweight people worldwide and the billions of people who experience bullying or sexual assault, transform their life positively thru JustHuynh Fitness' martial arts and power athletics training program.

Had I taken corporate career offers in 2016 after completing my MBA from Vanderbilt University and marrying my wife in Boston, "Ageless Athletic Assassin" would never have been written.

This book is for everyone who's experienced mental, physical, and fiscal pain from racism and discrimination from being short, fat, skinny, dumb, shy, weak, unathletic, and poor.

After reading "Ageless Athletic Assassin," I hope you thrive in life personally with your love, academically at an intellectual level, athletically as a fit fighter, and professionally to achieve your purpose in life.

www.justhuynh.com

Francis Huynh

STOP!

DO NOT READ THIS BOOK IF YOU CAN NOT HANDLE GETTING ON THE FITNESS FAST TRACK TO SUCCESS AND RATHER STAY STUCK ON THE TREADMILL OF MEDIOCRITY

CONTENTS

Chapter 4:
Overcoming Asian Discrimination

Chapter 5:
Asian Martial Arts Influences

Chapter 6:
JustHuynh Fitness Origins

Chapter 7:
Martial Arts For Life

Chapter 8:
Anti-Bullying Self Defense

Chapter 9:
Superhuman Warrior Skills

PART 2:
ATHLETIC (SUPERSTAR)

Chapter 10:
Global Obesity

Chapter 11:
Fitness Metrics

Chapter 12:
Killing Obesity 3 Times

Chapter 17:
90 Day Fitness Transformation

PART 3:
AGELESS (SUPERCENTENARIAN)

Chapter 18:
Decades of Dominant Ageing And Life

Chapter 19:
Supercentenarian Fitness Secrets

INTRODUCTION

By making the "Ageless Athletic Assassin" a healthy habit you will be able to live longer (Ageless), stay fit (Athletic), and defend yourself (Assassin) - allowing you to thrive personally and professionally. JustHuynh Fitness' program is built with the goal of transforming you with the principles of developing Olympic speed, lethal power, and life longevity where you can unleash the beast as your own "Superman" or "Wonder Woman."

Remember "Rome wasn't built in one day," meaning you will not undo years of unhealthy habits from one workout. You must be consistent to build your "Roman Empire" body, mind, and life.

Assassin is covered in Chapters 1-8. In Chapter 1 "You Only Live Once," you'll learn about why health is wealth, global obesity facts, how to live life purposefully, and about the three most important people in your life. In Chapter 2 "Fast Track to Success," you'll learn how to take action on your health today and make an impact in your community healthwise. In Chapter 3 "Bamboo Ceiling For Model Minorities," you'll learn about the pressures Asian Americans face as a Model Minority where parents emphasize the way to the American Dream is thru education but Asian Americans face racism and discrimination, referred to as the Bamboo Ceiling, of not being able to attain leadership positions in many phases of life from school to work to sports to politics. In Chapter 4 "Overcoming Asian Discrimination," you'll learn about how fitness saved me from committing suicide various times in life due to being discriminating against for being a perpetual Asian foreigner, fat, weak, and dumb. In Chapter 5 "Asian Martial Arts Influencers," you'll learn how martial arts founders developed self-defense techniques due to bullying and racism. In Chapter 6 "JustHuynh Fitness Origins," you'll learn how martial arts, track, the service industry, elite American universities, and Boston's winning culture contributed to the "just win" way of life. In Chapter 7 "Martial Arts For Life," you'll learn how martial arts helps women against rape, men against bullying, politicians (President Barack Obama), CEOs, Hollywood (Gal Gadot), singers (Wu Tang Clan), football defenders (Dallas Cowboys Doomsday Defense), basketball scorers (Kobe Bryant's Mamba Mentality from Bruce Lee), and soccer strikers (Zlatan Ibrahimovic) thrive in their lives. In Chapter 8 "Anti-Bullying Self Defense," you'll learn the benefits of self-defense against bullying and sexual assault. In Chapter 9 "Superhuman Warrior Skills," you'll learn the benefits of swimming, sprinting, and self-defense practiced by Super Soldiers in armies around the world -

especially human anatomy one-move kill shots and a 9-move combo to defend your life.

Athletic is covered in Chapters 10-17. In Chapter 10 "Global Obesity," you'll learn how to get motivation from sports around the world year-round to not be lazy and what is considered a dangerous waist size. In Chapter 11 "Fitness Metrics," you'll learn physical and mental fitness metrics, keys to athletic development, and physical fitness tests. In Chapter 12 "Slaying Obesity 3 times," you'll learn how I overcame childhood, college, and adult obesity. In Chapter 13 "Governments Fight Fat," you'll learn how countries like Finland made fitness publicly accessible, Japan holds companies accountable for their employee's health, London's junk food ad ban, and how to defeat bad actors in the sickness industry. In Chapter 14 "Coaching," you'll learn how coaching can take your life, health, and business to the next level. In Chapter 15 "Confidence and Mental Health," you'll learn how fitness can help you overcome suicidal thoughts, celebrity fitness transformations, and that fear is just a state of mind that can be overcome. In Chapter 16 "Habitual Commitment," you'll learn about mental preparation, how to make exercise fun, and common fitness money wasters to watch out for. In Chapter 17 "90 Day Fitness Transformation," you'll learn realistic weight loss goals based on calorie intake and exercise burn; and the benefits of weight lifting 3 times a week and performing cardio 3 times a week.

Ageless is covered in Chapters 18-23. In Chapter 18 "Decades of Dominant Ageing and Life," you'll learn how to dominate in fitness and business from your teenage years (Cardi B and Mark Zuckerberg) to when you reach 100 years old (The Queen Mother) for every 10 years of your life. In Chapter 19 "Supercentenarian Fitness Secrets," you'll learn the health secrets of Okinawa Japan (Land of Immortals), supercentenarian health habits, JustHuynh Fitness' signature bulletproof warm-up routine, and post workout recovery routines. In Chapter 20 "Time Wasters," you'll learn how to eliminate common time wasters such as social media, websites, gaming, online TV, and unproductivity at work (average 2 hours a day), can help you save up to the needed 1 hour a day for exercise. In Chapter 21 "Eat To Live," you'll learn how to approach your daily calorie intake, cautions when eating out, and ability to avoid unhealthy habits like alcohol, smoking, and drugs. In Chapter 22 "Love and Sex," you'll learn how exercise can help men with erectile dysfunction and women with sexual desire droughts, the benefits of self-love, and the benefits of sex as a form of exercise for your health. In Chapter 23 "Lucid Dreams," you'll learn how being able to positively dream and putting those dreams to action can accelerate your life.

PART I

ASSASSIN (SUPERHERO)

In any moment of decision, the best thing you can do is the right thing, the next best thing is the wrong thing, and the worst thing you can do is nothing

- Theodore Roosevelt

CHAPTER 1

YOU ONLY LIVE ONCE

Remembering that you are going to die is the best way I know to avoid the trap of thinking you have something to lose

- Steve Jobs

HEALTH IS WEALTH

In ancient Greece, physical strength, health, and beauty were central to one's excellence as were creative talent, intelligence, or moral character. Celebrities and leading business executives are part of a secretive world where food, exercise, vitamins, nutritional supplements, medical care, and ageing are mastered. They take their health seriously rather than wasting time on non-value add life activities. Rich or poor, you too can be proactive with your health instead of making excuses that you don't have time for exercise.

Famous Greek philosophers Socrates, Plato, and Aristotle all valued their health. In 468 BC, Plato's teacher Socrates said "No citizen has a right to be an amateur in the matter of physical training...what a disgrace it is for a man or woman to grow old without ever seeing the beauty and strength of which his or her body is capable." Here, Socrates wants you to know that you're doing a disservice to your life if you don't unlock your best physical form thru exercise. Greek philosopher Plato said "To succeed in life, perfection is achieved thru education + exercise." Plato reminds you to focus on your mind thru continuous learning and body thru exercise. Plato's student Aristotle said "We are what we repeatedly do. Excellence, then, is not an act, but a habit." In order to reach your best physical form, you need to make exercise a daily habit just like brushing your teeth.

Martial artists know the benefits of prioritizing health that can help you achieve your wealth goals. Imi Lichtenfeld, the Father of Krav Maga, had a life-changing quote in his book "Krav Maga: How to Defend Yourself Against Armed Assault" saying "Everyone wants to be in someone else's place: At the circus a young, muscular gymnast performs acrobatic feats on the trapeze, while in the audience below, in the most expensive seat, sits a rich, fat businessman with a cigar between his lips and a stunning girl on his arm. The businessman says to himself: "I would give all I have in order to be like him, young, athletics, without a care in the world," and the acrobat, who sees him from high up on the trapeze, thinks: "I wish I could be in his place, a rich man with such a beautiful woman, who can afford the most expensive seat at the circus and watch a young, poor, unfortunate guy like me endanger his life for a few cents." Like the Greek philosophers mentioned, you will thrive in life if sharpen both your body for health and your mind to achieve the wealth you need for an amazing life.

GLOBESITY - 2.2 BILLION OVERWEIGHT

"Globesity" a word first used by the World Health Organization (WHO) implying that the World is getting fat. Lack of fitness is now the leading cause of preventable death. Below are facts related to obesity in the United States:

- Obesity leads to diabetes, cancer, amputations, mental health issues, and even death
- Losing 7% of your body weight in as little as 3 months can improve your insulin performance by 57%
- In 2018 per the Centers for Disease Control and Prevention's (CDC) National Health Statistics Report, the average BMI for men was 29.1 and 29.6 for women. This is concerning as a healthy BMI is between 18.5 and 24.9. One is considered overweight with a BMI between 25 to 29.9 and obese with a BMI over 30. 66% of Americans are overweight and 33% of Americans are obese. Globally, 2.2 billion people are overweight and 400 million people have diabetes. There are more overweight people (2.2 billion) than the 600 million people worldwide who are starving for food
- Professionally, medical costs to care for patients with obesity are $210 billion per year in the United States. Obesity also affects companies where employees experience job absenteeism and lower productivity at work
- Obese adults have a 50-100% increased risk of premature death. The National Center for Chronic Disease Prevention and Health Promotion estimates 300,000 premature deaths from obesity each year

- Children learn lifestyle habits from their adult parents. Children with an obese parent have an 80% chance of becoming obese adults when they grow up
- 1/3 of cancer deaths are related to poor diet and lack of exercise
- 80% of people fail to meet WHO's Health Guideline of exercising 3 times per week
- 60% of new gym members, especially during the month of January for New Year's Fitness Resolutions, quit going to the gym 2 months after signing up.
- 80% of the 55 million Americans with gym memberships don't go to the gym
- People are often shy reaching out for help in the gym so go thru weight battles on their own - sometimes failing and dying
- Per the FBI crime clock, a violent crime is committed every 26.3 seconds - leading many citizens to learn unarmed and armed combat
- Per RAINN (Rape, Abuse, & Incest National Network), Americans are sexually assaulted every 98 seconds - leading to many self defense classes for men and women
- The U.S. Department of Health and Human Services as well as the World Health Organization recommends adults exercise at least 3 times per week to avoid health issues such as obesity, diabetes, cardiovascular disease, cancer, leg amputations, and even death

Behind these statistics are personal stories of needless suffering or death - not of strangers, but of family members, friends, even ourselves. Instead of exercising more and eating less, we are eating more and exercising less. To reach your target health via weight, the more you lose, the more of you there is - helping you contribute to your family, business, and community.

For the sake of humanity, cities around the world are spending taxpayer money on public fitness spaces such as running tracks, sports fields, and workout equipment within walking distance of your home - making it as convenient as possible to exercise in your neighborhood.

You spend the majority of your time at home and work. If you live in a luxury apartment or home, many developers provide a full-size gym as a wellness amenity to attract loyal tenants. All you need to do is go downstairs and use the gym.

For people who live in a home or apartment without a gym, you can deduct purchase of in-home gym equipment as a medical expense with a doctor's letter stating the equipment is a prescription for you to lose weight in treating obesity, diabetes, heart disease, or another health issue.

At work, many companies and commercial real estate developers invest in onsite gyms for employees to use as companies understand that a healthy workforce reduces healthcare costs and improves work productivity. With time as the most common excuse commuting to the gym, you can cancel your gym membership now with gyms available at your work and home.

Having personally overcome obesity 3 times (childhood, college, and adult), I never wanted to risk being morbidly obese ever again so started being proactive instead of reactive with my exercise and nutrition or end up being buried in a fat casket from premature death. Unlike smallpox which was virtually eliminated through vaccination - there is no vaccination for obesity and lack of fitness. As such, I realized that physical health is not a commodity to be bargained for, nor can it be swallowed in the form of drugs and pills. Health has to be earned through blood, sweat, and tears.

Thru personal experience, if I had continued staying fat, I would have suffered the same pain as the 2.2 billion overweight people - unable to actively play with your children, look great physically in public, get a great job as employers discreetly discriminate against fat people who are a large medical expense for companies, poor sex life, enjoy life functions such as fitting comfortable into an airplane seat without nearby passengers giving you disgusted stares, move around without losing your breathe, and stay away from sickcare (situation where you have to rely on the healthcare system for preventable medical issues thru exercise).

HOW I WENT FROM FAT TO FIT

Instead of being content with being made fun of as fat, dumb, and weak, I committed myself to be sexy, smart, and strong thru martial arts and power athletics in order to build the best body and mind to thrive in life personally and professionally.

By being fit at a young age just like it is beneficial to start investing young, you allow yourself to achieve your life goals thru blood, sweat, and tears such as obtaining an Ivy league level education (for me: Bowdoin, Vanderbilt), landing a dream job (for me: PwC, Samsung, FBI), courting a compatible love partner for the rest of your life (for me: Thao), and realizing your entrepreneurial calling and purpose in life (for me: JustHuynh Fitness).

After getting married in my hometown of South Portland, Maine and completing MBA from Vanderbilt University in 2016, I took the biggest risk of my life by turning down $100,000+ career opportunities with Samsung and the FBI to pursue my personal passion of launching a social fitness company that helps people JustHuynh "Just Win" at health by training together for the needed social accountability and motivation to achieve their fitness goals thru martial arts and power athletics. JustHuynh Fitness' mission is to help over 2 billion overweight people worldwide overcome obesity, mental health, and ageing issues - all of which I've worked extremely hard to conquer.

Before I was fat, I was a scrawny skinny Asian kid with the body type of a toothpick. My breakout from the toothpick body came at age 10 when I ate fast food and beef stew while drinking soda to go from skinny to fat.

This resulted in my first encounter with obesity as a child at age 10. These were tough times as I was made fun of for being fat, weak, slow, dumb, short, and Asian. I'm thankful that karate, track, and healthy eating helped me lose weight, gain confidence and become a champion in life.

Growing up watching Bruce Lee and Dragon Ball Z, my goal was to become the next great action star in Hollywood. One of my peak highlights was when I was a Karate blue belt matched up against a second degree black belt in a sparring fight. Having watched kung fu movies and repeating countermoves religiously while also scouting the black belt's fighting style, I went in for a sweep followed by a flying front kick - resulting in the black belt flying across the room. My karate master immediately stopped the match saying my knockout move was not karate and asked where I learned the move. Not nervous, I let my karate master know that the knockout move was learned from watching Kung Fu films. He respected my ability to incorporate techniques that work from other martial arts forms just as Bruce Lee did with Jeet Kune Do because you want to be formless when in combat to respond with various striking or defense techniques.

During my senior year in high school track, I was overconfident as best in the race so didn't stretch before the hurdle race. Going full speed resulted in straining my right hamstring followed by falling over the hurdle in which I smashed my face on the floor while my body slid - resulting in being unconscious for 10 minutes on the floor with the whole arena going silent. My mom, coach, and family came over in tears because they realized I forever lost my top speed from not stretching. I also had to deal with losing my right eyebrow for 2 months from my face sliding on the floor.

Depressed from losing my top speed, I stopped taking care of my health in college - drinking beer, eating pizza, and sitting on the couch watching TV which led to my second time being obese. It was tough being obese in a peer pressure bubble at a small college with only 1,600 students as I was not in shape and good looking compared to other guys which made it hard to make many friends as most college kids social lives are based around college athletics and weekend campus parties. Fortunately, some of my classmates were knowledgeable about weight lifting which was an important add-on to my existing knowledge of speed training. Speed training and weight lifting helped me overcome obesity a second time. So on an unfortunate day during my last year in college while playing flag football barefoot on grass, I stepped on a piece of glass from a broken beer bottle caused by a drunk college kid that forever altered the gait of my left foot. The human body only has 10 pints of blood and I lost 10% of my total blood (1 pint of blood) in seconds when I pulled the glass out of my foot where blood spurted out everywhere into surrounding friends faces like water out of a firehose before I went to the hospital.

Depressed once again after graduating college, I continued developing terrible health habits as a travelling management consultant resulting in my third time in life being obese. Averaging 200 nights a year away from home living in Starwood Hotels for 4 years straight, these 4 years were tough as the hotel gyms had limited fitness equipment and nutrition consisted of unhealthy meals and alcohol as consultants ate out every night with clients or the team until 10PM which didn't leave enough time for the unhealthy food to metabolize and made us too tired to workout with the limited gym equipment in the morning before work.

Health wasn't a priority until I went in for my annual health check-up at 22 years old weighing 160 pounds for a 5'2"guy which is obese on an Asian scale. Shocked with my annual health checkup, the health coach advised me to train with partners for the needed accountability and motivation in achieving my fitness goals because going alone as a lone wolf is tough.

What's ironic is that I already knew about all the fitness and nutrition knowledge the health coach provided. This is not uncommon because most people have the knowledge, but don't act on their knowledge such as me in my obese situation. I learned martial arts from my karate master and Chinese martial arts films. For power athletics, I learned the benefits of high intensity interval training from my high school track coach and weight lifting from my friends in college. What killed me was the lack of purpose in life. Realizing that being healthy would help me thrive personally to find a future wife, academically to excel at the highest levels intellectually, athletically by being the fittest athlete on the field given my size, and professionally to be the most valuable asset in an organization.

Training with partners helped me bring my weight down from 160 pounds to 140 pounds. My high school track coach said it best in one of his many memorable quotes saying "if you cheat now, you'll cheat later on your wives!" reminding me to never forget about my health again as health is the foundation for your wealth and life satisfaction.

In today's social media age of Instagram and photoshopped magazines of abs and butts, there's a lot of pressure for quick fixes such as yo-yo diets and plastic surgery to shift unwanted fat from your beer belly or jiggly arms to desirable places like your butt or breasts - with the hope of looking like Kim Kardashian or Channing Tatum. I'm proud to have gone from fat to fit naturally thru exercise and nutrition. You can as well.

Academically, I used to be a dumb underachieving student in school thus failing to meet the high standards that my parents set for me as a "Model Minority" which is the stereotype that Asian children are expected to be the top scholars in school especially in the STEM subjects of science, technology, engineering, and math. Being dumb was not pleasant as nobody wanted me on their team as my teammates would end up having to do extra work to clean up my mistakes. Being dumb also led to struggles in real life where I couldn't have an intelligent conversation with others on various topics.

Numerous studies show that exercise enhances cognitive function. As a result, I went from an underachieving middle school student to graduating in the top ten of my high school class with a 4.0 GPA - gaining admission into one of the most prestigious American liberal arts colleges in 4th ranked Bowdoin College in my home state of Maine whose successful alumni include American Civil War hero Joshua Chamberlain, 14th President of the United States Franklin Pierce, Netflix Founder Reed Hastings, Subway Founder Peter Buck, L.L. Bean Chairman Leon Gorman, former AMEX CEO Ken Chenault, Barclays CEO Jes Staley, legendary hedge fund manager Stanley Druckenmiller, U.S. Senate Majority Leader George Mitchell, and 43rd Mayor of San Francisco Ed Lee. This was a big deal in my family as I'm the first in family to graduate from college as my parents came over to the United States as boat people from Vietnam after the Vietnam War. The difficult backstory is that most Vietnamese boat people were sponsored to warmer states Vietnamese communities such as Orange County California, Falls Church Virginia, or Dallas Texas but my family ended up in cold Maine - sponsored by Priest Father Donald Gilbert. Acclimating to life in Maine as Asian Americans was difficult as Maine is the whitest state in America with a population that is 95% white and 1% Asian.

After 4 years as a management consultant - living in hotels on average 200 nights per year racking up the highest levels of airline (Delta) and hotel status (Starwoods) like George Clooney in the movie "Up in the Air," I wanted to work internally instead of externally for an innovative company or pursue my entrepreneurial passion for fitness. To do this, I applied and got admitted into Vanderbilt University for my MBA (Masters of Business Administration) - the fittest and brightest university in the world.

In terms of being the fittest, Vanderbilt University competes in the Southeastern Conference (SEC) which is regarded as the most accomplished sports conference in the United States for winning 43 national football championships and 21 basketball championships - featuring elite athletic universities Alabama, Tennessee, Georgia, LSU, Auburn, Florida, Texas A&M, Ole Miss, South Carolina, and Kentucky. Vanderbilt University is recognized for producing many notable professionals in baseball and football. The best Vanderbilt University baseball athletes are David Price ($217 million 7-year contract with the Boston Red Sox, #1 Pick in 2007 MLB Draft) and Walker Buehler (Winning Pitcher in the Los Angeles Dodgers one victory against 2018 World Series Champion Boston Red Sox, #24 Pick in 2015 MLB Draft). The best basketball players included Darius Garland (#8 Projected Pick in 2019 NBA Draft). The best football players are Jay Cutler ($126 million 7-year contract with the Chicago Bears, #11 Pick in 2006 NFL Draft), Casey Hayward ($36 million 3-year contract with Los Angeles Chargers for making Pro Bowl 2 times), and Jordan Matthews (Set numerous SEC Wide Receiver records, #42 Pick in 2014 NFL Draft).

In terms of brightest per U.S. News ranking, Vanderbilt University is ranked #14 best University in the United States. The most successful alumni are Hospital Corporation of America (HCA) CEO Thomas Frist Jr., Ingram Family of Ingram Industries (Martha Rivers Ingram, John R. Ingram, Orrin H. Ingram II, David B. Ingram), Dollar General CEO Cal Turner Jr., Bain & Company founder Bill Bain, Boston Consulting Group Founder Bruce Henderson, NASDAQ CEO Adena Friedman, American Airlines CEO Doug Parker, 45th Vice President of the United States Al Gore, and Jack Daniel's President J. Reagor Motlow.

At Vanderbilt, I felt energized in a campus full of athletic Wonder Woman and Superman with super high IQs. Professionally, I took my business knowledge to the next level by studying entrepreneurship, operations, and strategy. I applied my new knowledge with Sprint in Kansas as an internal consultant after my 1st year of MBA to optimize employee talent. After graduating in 2016, I worked in Samsung's customer service division focused on the customer journey from awareness to retention.

I transformed to peak fitness over these two years - having 100% control of my nutrition and committing myself to 4:44AM workouts 6 times a week. I've always enjoyed social fitness in organizing group workouts to help people with accountability and motivation. At Bowdoin, I organized the most diverse intramural basketball team in history named "Just Put It In," a pun for putting the basketball thru the net, to win the school championship - we had two tall white centers in Rob Stanley and Grant Easterbrook, two sharp shooting black forwards in Jarrod Powell and David Paul, and three speedy Asian guards in Toni Kong, my brother Brian, and myself. Our biggest moment in the playoffs was when I drained a deep 3-point shot over a kid while he tried to rattle me by screaming "You can't shoot you short Asian kid!" He was dejected and loss face when we humbly celebrated our win.

As a management consultant on the road away, I organized 4:44AM morning workouts and evening basketball or soccer games to boost team camaraderie and stay healthy. At Vanderbilt, I organized the first ever graduate school olympics where future business leaders (MBAs), lawyers (JDs), and doctors (MDs) battled each other once a year to claim status as the fittest graduate school program in competitions on the track, soccer fields, and swimming pool. MBAs are typically 28 years old compared to JDs and MDs who are 22 years old so it was extremely satisfying to defeat the younger athletes to prove that "age is just a number." It's how well you eat and exercise that matters. After graduating and getting married in 2016, I moved back up to Boston and continued organizing social fitness events by partnering with the City of Boston in it's annual Social Fitness Festival that brings the city together for all sorts of workouts ranging from martial arts (JustHuynh Fitness), dancing, cycling, and boot camps.

On a personal level, I met my wife in Boston who has supported me thru my health struggles with obesity and stayed strong during our long-distance relationships from consulting and business school. With a successful career post-MBA and marriage, my wife supported me in taking the biggest risk of our lives to pursue my passion to improve the health of the over 2 billion people worldwide thru martial arts and power athletics program with our JustHuynh Fitness company. This was not easy, as I could have easily settled into a corporate desk job with a $120,000 annual stable paycheck to start a family. Instead, I chose to go thru the entrepreneurial journey where you're fighting just to put food on the table and making rent as startups are not all unicorn stories like you read about in the news. Not wanting to waste my life in jobs that I don't wake up in the morning excited for, I turned down 6 figure career opportunities from 2 of the most respected and powerful brands in the world - FBI and Samsung.

In business, being "fit" is a "lead magnet" in meeting people outside of your normal circle, where you then use your IQ to "seal the deal" as customers confirm that you are the best solution for their needs by happily opening their wallets to you as you solve their pain.

With my track record of success overcoming obesity by making health a habit just like brushing my teeth, I've grown my personal brand and known by friends and colleagues as "franchise," "special agent," "super saiyan," "4:44AM," "the closer," "assassin," and "ninja."

LEGACY - FIND YOUR CALLING

There's something coming for all of us. It's called death. Rather than fearing death, death can become one of our greatest counselors. So, if this was the last week of your life, what would you cherish most? How would you live? How would you love? What truth would you tell today?

From birth to death, you'll have many life-changing moments: graduating top of high school class, admissions into an elite college, landing your dream job, earning your first paycheck, getting down on one knee to propose to your girlfriend or being the girlfriend who says "yes!," exchanging rings during your wedding ceremony, seeing your first-born child, changing the life of your first customer as an entrepreneur, delivering the eulogy at parent's funeral, seeing your children graduate college, seeing your children get married, becoming a grandparent, celebrating your 60th birthday, and being recognized for your contributions to society by family and friends.

In David Graeber's book "Bullshit Jobs," David wants to help you not remain stuck in bullshit jobs (i.e. I know friends in $100,000 jobs where a typically 8 hour day is spent sending 2 emails so the rest of the day is spent swiping on Tinder, playing video games, online shopping, napping, scrolling social media, and watching online TV shows), which he says is 50% of all jobs. Bullshit jobs have no value to the world or company and more importantly no value to you since you're earning a paycheck for meaningless work like the character Big Head does in the "Silicon Valley" series.

David Graeber's message about "Bullshit Jobs" goes hand-in-hand with Elon Musk's advice on his reason for being an entrepreneur saying "To be useful for other people. Make things that people love. Maximize probability that the future is exciting." More importantly, Elon loves entrepreneurship because like sports (i.e. Michael Jordan, Serena Williams, LeBron James) and entertainment (i.e. Taylor Swift, Ellen DeGeneres, Dwayne Johnson, Gal Gadot, Kim Kardashian), your worth in society is based on your merit of serving customers instead of restricting your income potential climbing the corporate ladder where salary raises and promotions are based on tenure and winning office politics against your peer rival co-workers. At MIT's Commencement Address in 2017, Apple CEO Tim Cook gave advice to the college graduates saying "Use your minds and hands — and your hearts — to build something bigger than yourselves." Imagine how advanced society would be with 1 million Elon Musk instead of 1 million average Joes.

Death can give anyone a wakeup call. I've had my share of near death experiences skydiving from 15,000 feet over the Great Barrier Reef in Australia, bungy jumping from a 17 story (50 meters) high platform in Australia, nearly drowning while swimming in the deep open water of Bondi Beach in Australia, made a Citizen's arrest of a mentally-ill lady tagging behind my friend and I with a knife, driving away at high speed in a taxi from a gang fight during our family trip in La Boca Argentina, avoiding the violent 2016 Olympic Protestors from the favelas in Rio de Janeiro Brazil, ducking away from a potential knife attack at night when my brother and I ran a family errand near Iguazu Falls in Argentina, losing a pint of blood from pulling out glass from my foot, blacking out for 10 minutes after tripping over a hurdle at full speed, and many more.

Having survived so many near-death experiences, I channel Steve Jobs view of life "Remembering that you are going to die is the best way I know to avoid the trap of thinking you have something to lose." Steve didn't want to wake up disgruntled like most people so pursued his passion of "making a dent in the universe" where he was able to go home at night and happily say "What a great life." Steve's early death left a legacy for all to remember. Watch his funeral event online so you get inspired to pursue your passion as life is too short to "check the box" for an unsatisfying paycheck. An example of Steve influencing people with his "everyone dies so there's nothing to lose" philosophy is when Steve famously lured John Sculley, the PepsiCo president, to run Apple by saying "Do you want to spend the rest of your life selling sugared water or do you want a chance to change the world?" After Steve's death, he remains the guiding light for many entrepreneurs as they can relate to him as misfits, disruptors, game-changers, and rebels.

To put life into perspective as your time alive is limited - the oldest person to ever live was 122-year-old Jeanne Calment, ask yourself 3 questions: What do I stand for? What do I want my life to be about? What do I want people to say when I die? My legacy is for JustHuynh Fitness to help people live long happily, overcome bullying, and boost confidence thru martial arts and power athletics.

THE THIRD PLACE - 3 IMPORTANT PEOPLE

The majority of your life is spent at home, work, and gym. In each of these places are the three most important people in your life: your wife/husband at home, your boss/customer at work, and your fitness trainer in the gym. I live by the saying "Dominate the exercise room in order to dominate the bedroom and boardroom."

In your first place at home, your wife or husband serves as your friend for life in keeping you in check especially in the darkest of times so that you can be saved from potential suicidal thoughts that many lonely people have when they face hardships especially financial and social pressure.

In your second place at work, if you're an employee, making your boss look good helps you earn your paycheck to pay the bills. If you're an entrepreneur CEO, your job is to provide the best solution to your customers in order for your business to thrive as customers pick winners with their wallet.

JustHuynh Fitness' mission is to be the third place that keeps you healthy thru martial arts and power athletics so you can dominate at home personally and at work professionally. If you truly commit yourself with our program, you will be more confident, gain self defense capabilities and enjoy a long-living life. Our instructors online and in-studio will provide you the most comfortable environment where you'll be able to unlock your unlimited potential. Just like your daily interaction with your wife/husband and boss/customers, your daily interaction with our instructors will be one of the most important as we can guide you in moments of stress.

CHAPTER 2

FAST TRACK TO SUCCESS

Ask people to forgive your greatness, not permission to be great

- Francis Huynh

CONGRATULATIONS FOR MAKING IT HERE

You can continue to be stuck on the treadmill of mediocrity or jump on the fast track to success. If you're satisfied with mediocrity, please STOP READING as you should go back to whatever else is more important than your HEALTH.

Diet is easy - just smash your large plates for portion control and eat well-balanced meals with protein, vegetables, and fat. Cut the carbs, booze, sugar, fast food, and smoking. Keep you daily calorie intake at 1,500 for women and 1,800 for men.

Exercise is the most difficult piece of the health puzzle because a time commitment to get off the couch is required. You should remember that insanity is expecting greatness from doing the same thing - so you won't be able to burn calories while watching TV, using social media, and pursuing unhealthy habits such as drinking alcohol.

SHARE BOOK WITH LOVED ONES

I've dedicated my life to write this book for you and would be grateful if you could review this book on Amazon and upload a selfie picture of you with this book on Instagram, Linkedin, Facebook, and Twitter (Weibo, Linkedin, and WeChat if you live in China) using the hashtag #agelessathleticassassin and #justhuynhfitness tagging @justhuynh_ and @franciskhuynh.

SWEATWORKING SPEAKING EVENT

If your community, event, city, or workplace would like a motivational cardio-burning event to get healthy, I'd love to come conduct a 45-minute workout and hold a Q&A session for a minimum 250 person attendance. You can book me at www.justhuynh.com/speaking

FITNESS TRANSFORMATION JOURNEY

Get started or take your fitness to the next level with JustHuynh Fitness' martial arts and power athletics training program online at www.justhuynh.com. The online training program will guide you thru 3 cardio (martial arts) and 3 power athletics (strength training) workouts each week. JustHuynh Fitness currently has studios where you can work on cardio together in your community. If your community doesn't currently have a nearby studio and you'd like one nearby, you can sign-up to be a potential licensee of the JustHuynh Fitness program by opening a studio in your area by filling out a contact form online at www.justhuynh.com/become-a-licensee.

To keep yourself accountable, post a selfie from each workout onto Instagram or Weibo using the hashtag #agelessathleticassassin and #justhuynhfitness tagging @justhuynh_ and @franciskhuynh.

COMMUNITY LEADER

Give the gift of leadership by letting your community know about JustHuynh Fitness' martial arts and power athletics program at www.justhuynh.com. You can contact your local/state/federal government, health insurance company, college alma mater, gym's wellness director, apartment gym manager, influencers, and local news channels about joining and referring our program with your family and friends.

JOIN THE JUSTHUYNH TEAM

If you're a martial artist with at least 2 years of formal martial arts training who would love to be a part of the JustHuynh Fitness team conducting group fitness classes, please apply at www.francishuynh.com/instructor.

If you're interested in becoming a licensee of the JustHuynh Fitness program by opening a studio in your area in our mission to be in all major cities in the world, please fill out a contact form online at www.justhuynh.com/become-a-licensee.

If you're interested in partnering with JustHuynh Fitness to help your community with self defense and confidence, reach out to us at www.francishuynh.com/contact.

CHAPTER 3

BAMBOO CEILING FOR MODEL MINORITIES

Most convictions get wiped after a period of time. But there's no way of erasing what happened in July 2015. The word 'racist' is a permanent stain against my name. It's worse than a criminal record. It's on YouTube when my kids type in their dad's name and it comes up 'Jamie Vardy racist.' On Google, too. It's horrible

- Jamie Vardy (Leicester City Striker on verbally abusing Asian casino player three times)

LACK OF ASIAN ROLE MODELS AT THE TOP

America is the land of opportunity where everyone from all races can get a fair shot of achieving their dream career goals in business, politics, sports, Hollywood, music, showbiz, comedy, and more. Unfortunately Asian Americans lack role models who are the most recognized and top earners in their profession. This is called the "Bamboo Ceiling" where Asians are the most educated ethnic group "Model Minority" but don't hold the top positions or are the highest paid in their professions due to racism and stereotypes that Asians are weak, shy, and incapable of leading. In business, there are lack of Fortune 500 CEOs like Jeff Bezos. In politics, Asian Americans hope to break the minority ceiling like Barack Obama did by becoming the first African American President of the United States of America. In athletics, Asian Americans don't have a global icon like Michael Jordan to look up to. On the big screen, Asians don't have a Dwayne Johnson whose movies consistently make more than $100 million at the box office. In music, Asians don't have superstars like Taylor Swift and Jay Z. In showbiz, Asians dream of being able to connect with TV audiences like Oprah Winfrey and Ellen DeGeneres. To make people laugh, Asians hope for role models like Jerry Seinfeld and Kevin Hart.

Francis Huynh

There are one-hit wonders every now and then, but Asian Americans need a pipeline talent of industry dominance to inspire future generations. Growing up in school, work, or sports, I was always viewed as the "trophy Asian" meaning I was there to "check the box" so the particular organization looked good for considering my talent based on the color of my skin. All professions should be open to promoting diverse talent instead of being narrow minded by only focusing on talent from specific races based on their skin color and stereotypes. For example in basketball, Asian American Jeremy Lin had a great month of basketball in 2012 with the New York Knicks so people called the event "Linsanity." Such performances are common for LeBron James and Kobe Bryant with nobody calling a good month from them "BronSanity" or "KobeMania." This proves that people are surprised when Asians do something great in America.

Instead of 1 million average Joes, imagine if the world has 1 million Jeff Bezos, 1 million Taylor Swifts, 1 million Barack Obamas, 1 million Serena Williams or 1 million Dwayne Johnsons. Society would thrive at an extremely rapid pace. Sadly, Asians don't have Asian role models they can hang in their bedroom for inspiration like non-Asians do to succeed in America at the highest level.

America shouldn't wait until year 2045 to start promoting talent from all ethnicities as the United States 2017 Census confirms the importance of racial minorities for the nation's future growth as the United States will become "minority white" in year 2045 where Whites will comprise 49.7% of the population compared to 24.6% for Hispanics, 13.1% for blacks, 7.9% for Asians, and 3.8% for multiracial populations. Since minorities as a group are younger than Whites, the minority White tipping point comes earlier for younger age groups where minority youth under 18 years old will outnumber Whites in 2020 and minorities age 18-29 will outnumber Whites in 2027. Thus, it is extremely important to invest in the nation's diverse youth and young adults now.

It saddens me when I hear people telling me and other Asian Americans to "go back to your country in Asia" because as a United States Citizen or Resident, Asian Americans too have the should have the same dignity as non-Asians to pursue the American Dream regardless of the color of our skin. Unfortunately, non-Asians continue to put down Asian Americans. Having personally survived 30 years of racism for being Asian, I'm most fearful for my children and will do my best as a father to culturally educate all communities that they interact with. People have to imagine if they were in "our Asian American shoes." How would your mental state be if you were brought down by racist remarks? As an offender, how would you sleep at night? Would your mom, dad, guardians, and family be proud that you're a racist? I'm a firm believer in equal opportunity where people of all races get considered and rewarded based on merit, not on skin color.

Prominent African American civil rights leaders have paved the way for minorities in America. Regarding race, Nelson Mandela said "No one is born hating another person because of the color of his skin or his background or his religion" meaning humans of all skin colors should be treated fairly. Regarding the use of violence to resolve confrontations, Martin Luther King Jr. said "Nonviolence is a powerful and just weapon. Which cuts without wounding and ennobles the man who wields it. It is a sword that heals. Nonviolence means avoiding not only external physical violence but also internal violence of spirit. You not only refuse to shoot a man, but you refuse to hate him. Returning hate for hate multiplies hate, adding deeper darkness to a night already devoid of stars. Darkness cannot drive out darkness; only light can do that. Hate cannot drive out hate; only love can do that." Regarding treating everyone as a human, Thurgood Marshall, the first African American U.S. Supreme Court member, said "In recognizing the humanity of our fellow beings, we pay ourselves the highest tribute."

RACISM FROM CHILD TO ADULT

For some reason, people think it is socially acceptable to make fun of Asians mainly because Asians are quiet and tend not to fight back. According to the FBI, "Asian Americans are attractive targets for violent crime due to racial stereotypes that paint Asians as submissive, compliant, and physically weak. In addition, linguistic barriers and a mistrust of law enforcement cause many Asian American victims to stay silent. Most alarming is that police often fail to report hate crimes on Asian Americans." Ex-con Ananza Emenike confirms this in his "Inside the Mind of a Criminal" interview saying "I choose Asian victims based on the assumptions that they carry a lot of cash, won't fight back, and won't go to police due to a language barrier."

As a newborn until grade 8, Asian Americans face racism and bullying in school. In high school, affirmative action proposals such as that in New York City complaining about "too many Asians" testing well on entrance exams has created an imbalance to African Americans and Hispanics. Rejecting talented Asian Americans at elite high schools to fulfill "race quotas" is racial discrimination. In high school, it's exciting to see states such as former Florida Governor Rick Scott creating a stipend for students experiencing racism and bullying to transfer to a different school so they can safely pursue their dreams thru an elite college.

In college, Asian Americans experience racism and bullying if they take up too much of the library for studying. At parties, teams, student clubs, or social events, Asian Americans can be left out because of their accent or introvertedness instead of their classmates welcoming them in. This makes for a miserable 4 years that should be the "best 4 years" of a young person's life. According to Eliza Noh, assistant professor of Asian-American studies at California State University-Fullerton, Asian American college students are 1.6 times more likely than non-Asians to make a serious suicide attempt.

As adults, Hollywood has painted Asian Americans as people who are good at math, tech savvy, shy, speak broken English, and weak. This makes it difficult for Asian American men and women to healthily succeed in life personally when they're trying to find love and professionally when they're held back from executive positions.

SOCIAL CREDIT SYSTEM

To reward and punish social behavior, China will be implementing a "Social Credit System" in year 2020 with punishments such as banning misbehaving citizens from flying or traveling on train, throttling your internet speed, banning you and your kids from the best schools, preventing you from getting the best jobs, keeping you out of the best hotels, confiscating your pets, and being publicly shamed as a bad citizen while well-behaved citizens earn rewards ranging from energy bill discounts, lower interest on bank loans, and better matches on dating websites.

Everyone especially celebrities with over 1 million followers on social media platforms such as Instagram, Twitter, and Weibo have a responsibility to act well as millions of followers mimic their behaviors. A racist post by a celebrity may mislead their social media followers to believe that it is socially acceptable to be racist to particular minority groups such as Asian Americans. Along the lines of the social credit system, anyone including celebrities should be publicly shamed for being a racist by calling out misbehaving celebrities on social media or celebrities will continue misusing their social platform.

Examples of publicly shamed celebrities are Mark Wahlberg for his 1988 racially motivated assault of beating down a Vietnamese man and soccer star Jamie Vardy who engaged in a racist outburst against an Asian man at a casino in 2015.

AMERICA'S FIRST ASIAN PRESIDENT

President Barack Obama paved the way for future African Americans who aspire to become President. Hillary Clinton (first female presidential candidate nominated by a major party - Democrat), Madeleine Albright (first female to become Secretary of State), Nancy Pelosi (first female Speaker of the United States House of Representatives), Rebecca Latimer Felton (first female United States Senator), Alexandria Ocasio-Cortez (youngest women ever elected to Congress at age 29), and Sandra Day O'Connor (first female to serve on United States Supreme Court) inspired women to attain the highest political positions. Today, Asian Americans don't have a role model who has become the first Asian American President of the United States of America.

In the United States Senate, only 3 out of 100 (3%) Senators are Asian - Mazie Hirono of Hawaii is Japanese, Tammy Duckworth of Illinois is Thai, and Kamala Harris of California is Afro-Asian. In the United House of Representatives, only 15 of 435 (3.4%) representatives are Asian Americans.

It is difficult for Asian Americans to attain the highest level in politics such as being the first Asian American President as racism is rampant at lower positions as experienced by former Labor Secretary Elaine Chao (first Asian-American woman to serve in a presidential cabinet when President George W. Bush appointed her Secretary of Labor in 2001) who is the wife of Senate Republican Leader Mitch McConnell. In defending his wife Elaine, Senator Mitch publicly shamed the racists for criticizing the Asian heritage of his wife saying "Elaine Chao is a shining example of the American dream: salt-of-the-earth folks who escaped oppression, came here with nothing, joined our great melting pot, worked exceptionally hard to build a thriving business, and then dedicated so much of their lives to giving back...It is unconscionable that anyone would use blatant race-baiting for political gain."

In 2018, former Massey Energy CEO Don Blankenship, a Republican from West Virginia, was criticized as racist for an ad attack towards Senate Majority Leader Mitch McConnell for growing rich from his "China family" saying "Swamp captain Mitch McConnell has created millions of jobs for China people. In fact, his China family has given him tens of millions of dollars." Upset, thirty-five Asian American groups across the United States called on the DNC and RNC to reject all future racist campaign rhetoric. The Asian Americans Advancing Justice (AAAJ) said "Asian Americans Advancing Justice is outraged and exasperated that once again, as midterm elections start to heat up, a candidate for elected office believes that saying blatant racist statements is appropriate. This most recent ad is yet another example in a long line of political advertising used to incite animosity or race-based fear of Asian Americans and other communities of color. It is clear this ad uses the myth of Asians being perpetual foreigners as a way to raise fear and concern. This is the same kind of tactic that led to shameful moments in U.S. history such as the Chinese Exclusion Act of 1882 and the incarceration of Japanese Americans during World War II. Americans have had enough of this stereotyping and fear-mongering. We reject these racist remarks. America and Americans are better than this." National Council of Asian Pacific Americans director Greg Orton said "It's campaign season again and disappointingly we find ourselves responding to more racism and xenophobia in political ads. This has to stop. The truth is that when racist or xenophobic language is used by any political party, it is painfully personal for that community, and in context to the AAPI community, reinforces the damaging narrative that we are 'outsiders' to the civic engagement process."

After returning from Vietnam as a prisoner of war, Senator John McCain continued to call his Vietnamese captors "gooks" then apologized saying "Out of respect to a great number of people whom I hold in very high regard, I will no longer use the term that has caused such discomfort. I deeply regret any pain I have caused. I apologize and renounce all language that is bigoted and offensive." Even though Senator McCain experienced great pain as a prisoner, he recognized that he shouldn't use racist references to his former captors so demonstrated maturity by apologizing.

In 2018, Republican Tom MacArthur in New Jersey's 3rd District was accused of sending a racist political mailer in New Jersey towards Democrat Andy Kim that used the chop suey font when referencing Asian American opponent Andy Kim and used imagery of fish markets common in Chinatown. Backed by public support, Andy Kim won the race becoming New Jersey's first Asian-American congressman despite his opponent's racist tactics.

In 2018, Republican Chris Collins in New York was deemed racist by Democrat Chinese-American from California Ted Lieu for an ad against Collins' Democratic opponent, Nate McMurray, speaking Korean, with subtitles saying his goal was to ship jobs overseas when he was a lawyer in Korea. The subtitles did not match what McMurray was saying in the video and there was a portrait of North Korean Kim Jong-Un. Ted told Collins to "Take your racist ad and shove it. You are an embarrassment to the House of Representatives. For folks who get angry after watching the racist ad, go to @Nate_McMurray website at votemcmurray.com and help Nate." Collins narrowly won - benefiting from the racist ads.

In Miami Florida, Miami Mayor Joe Carollo compared City Commissioner Ken Russell's hair to North Korean leader Kim Jong-un's saying "The more I look at you, I'm becoming fond of Kim Jong-un... I was just wondering if your Kim-like haircut is in favor or in protest of the nuclear negotiations with Trump and Kim." Russell, who is Japanese American, decried the joke as racist on Twitter saying "Tonight at City Commission, Commissioner Carollo made a joke likening my appearance to Korean dictator Kim Jong Un...I let him know that racist humor is unacceptable. People have made Asian jokes around me since I was a kid. Wasn't funny then. Not funny now."

In Detroit Michigan, African American Bettie Cook Scott and Asian American Stephanie Chang were running for the state Senate. Unfortunately, Bettie made racist remarks to Stephanie referring to her as "ching-chang" and the ching-chong." Bettie also called Stephanie's Asian American volunteers an "immigrant" saying "you don't belong here" and "I want you out of my country." Furthermore Bettie attacked Asian American Stephanie Chang's husband Sean Gray who is African American saying "I'm disgusted seeing black people hold signs for these Asians and not supporting their own people...you are a fool for marrying Chang." This was a personal attack to African American husband Sean Gray who responded saying "I asked Bettie not to speak about my wife in that manner." A friend of Stephanie who's an African American woman says "As an African-American woman, I've been called the N-word before in my life and you never forget it...Each time it's shocking and appalling and disgusting, so when you hear someone that's a minority and a woman using slurs against another minority that's a woman, it's just mind boggling and it just felt dirty." As a result Bettie apologized saying "I deeply regret the comments I made that have proven harmful to so many. Those are words I never should have said. I humbly apologize to Representative Chang, her husband, Mr. Gray, and to the broader Asian American community for those disparaging remarks. In the divisive age we find ourselves in, I should not contribute further to that divisiveness. I pray she and the Asian American community can find it in their hearts to forgive me." Let's hope Bettie's apology is not just lip service but a new sense of respect for people of all racial backgrounds.

In California #metoo activist California Assemblywoman Cristina Garcia was reprimanded by former Assembly Speaker John Perez in 2014 for making racially insensitive comments directed toward Asians when she lost a bill to Asian American community activists. Garcia also acknowledged using homophobic slurs including the word "faggot" aimed at Perez, the first openly gay speaker of the California State Assembly. This is in addition to being accused of groping a staff at a softball game and sexually harassing a male staff member after a night of drinking.

In Minnesota, Jennifer Carnahan is the first minority and first female elected to run the Republican Party of Minnesota. Born in South Korea and adopted by Minnesota parents Jennifer wrote a Facebook post about facing sexism and racism saying that "Some Republican Party leaders/executive committee members around this state have made racist comments about me, calling me 'dragon lady, a chink, a stupid Asian not even born in America and other awful racial slurs.

From city to State to national political positions, Asian Americans continue to experience racism that takes a toll on everyone mentally as they strive to dedicate their life to public service.

FORTUNE 500 CEOS - 0 EAST ASIANS

According to 2010 data from the U.S. Department of Labor, Asians are better educated than non-Asian races with more Asians age 25 and older having graduated college (52%) than white people of the same age (32%) yet Asians are underrepresented in leadership positions - a phenomenon referred to as the "bamboo ceiling." Asian Americans don't have role models CEOs or executives like Caucasians do with Jeff Bezos of Amazon, Steve Jobs of Apple, Warren Buffett of Berkshire Hathaway; Sara Blakely of Spanx, Abigail Johnson of Fidelity Investments, Mark Zuckerberg, Sheryl Sandberg, Dustin Moskovitz, Eduardo Saverin, Jan Koum, Brian Acton, Kevin Systrom, Mike Krieger, and Winklevoss Twins of Facebook; Jack Dorsey of Twitter; Evan Spiegel of Snapchat, Reed Hastings of Netflix; Brian Chesky, Joe Gebbia, and Nathan Blecharczyk of Airbnb; Travis Kalanick and Garrett Camp of Uber; Adam Neumann and Miguel McKelvey of WeWork; Larry Ellison of Oracle, Marc Benioff of Salesforce, Michael Bloomberg of Bloomberg; Larry Page, Sergey Brin, and Eric Schmidt of Google; Walton Family of Walmart, Phil Knight of Nike, Michael Dell of Dell; Bill Gates, Paul Allen, and Steve Ballmer of Microsoft; Elon Musk of Tesla, Ray Dalio of Bridgewater Associates, Jim Simons of Renaissance Technologies, Carl Icahn of Icahn Capital Management, Steve Cohen of Point72 Asset Management, David Tepper of Appaloosa Management, and Stephen A. Schwarzman of Blackstone Group.

Out of the CEOs in Fortune 500 companies, there are only 3 (.6%) with Asian CEOs - Satya Nadella of Microsoft, Sundar Pichai of Google, and

Shantanu Narayen of Adobe - who are all Indian Americans. If you're non-Indian American such as Japanese, Chinese, Korean, and Vietnamese, you have no Fortune 500 role model CEO in corporate America. As evident by the Fortune 500 CEO list, Asian Americans have the lowest chance of rising to executive management positions when compared with Whites, African Americans, and Hispanics in spite of having the highest educational attainment.

In Silicon Valley where entry level computer programmers are rewarded $250,000 at Facebook right out of college, Asians represent a small percentage of upper management and board positions. Statistics show that despite 33% of all software engineers in Silicon Valley being Asian, Asians make up only 6% of board members and 10% of corporate officers at the 25 largest companies in Silicon Valley.

Cultural values may also contribute to the disconnect between Asians and leadership in the U.S. Wesley Yang wrote in "New York" magazine "Western society teaches that "the squeaky wheel gets the grease" while Eastern society teaches that "the nail that sticks out gets hammered down."" Because of this, Eastern society groups are subject to "model minority" stereotypes being viewed as math geniuses, non-confrontational, submissive, and antisocial. In the workforce, some of these perceptions may seem positive in the short-term, but in the long-term they impede progression up the corporate ladder because upper management ignores evaluating Asian talent due to the stereotypes.

Asians are also discriminated due to their physical attributes such as being non-white, short, unfashionable, and weak because Asian don't fit the leadership prototype of being a tall white male. Discrimination from physical attributes combined with common stereotypes of Asian Americans as nerds, short, not good-looking, and socially inept create the "bamboo ceiling" that hold back Asian Americans from CEO positions.

In 2017, Silicon Valley Tech Company Palantir was fined $1.7 million to settle a government lawsuit for discriminating against Asian applicants. The labor department said that Palantir used a discriminatory hiring process in which Asian applicants were routinely eliminated in the resume screen and telephone interview phases despite being as qualified as white applicants. From a pool of 1,160 qualified software engineer applicants in which 85% were Asian, Palantir ended up hiring 14 non-Asian employees and only 11 Asian people.

In 1982, 27 year old Vincent Chin, a Chinese American, was brutally beaten to death with a baseball bat while being racial abused in Detroit by

Chrysler plant supervisor Ebens and his laid-off stepson Nitz outside a local bar 8 days before Vincent Chin's wedding. The killers blamed Chin because Japanese auto imports led to the decline of Detroit's Big Three saying "It's because of you little motherf*****s that we're out of work" despite the fact that Vincent is Chinese, not Japanese. Ebens and Nitz were ordered to pay $3,000 and serve three years probation, with no jail time. The lenient verdict led to protests from Asian-Americans with Detroit Chinese Welfare Council President saying "The ruling of Vincent's murder amounted to a $3,000 license to kill Chinese-Americans." Vincent's ruling supports the idea that Asian Americans are not treated as full citizens or "perpetual foreigners." Vincent's mom Lily Chin stated "What kind of law is this? What kind of justice? This happened because my son is Chinese. If two Chinese killed a white person, they must go to jail, maybe for their whole lives...Something is wrong with this country."

Although Asians haven't taken action on "bamboo ceiling" discrimination in the workplace, women in California have taken legal action on the "glass ceiling" that women face against men in executive and board positions of public companies. In 2018, California became the first state in the United States to require women be included on company boards of directors when Governor Jerry Brown signed the SB826 bill into law. The bill mandates that all publicly traded California companies have at least one woman on their boards by the end of 2019. By 2021, five-member boards will be expected to have two female members and boards with more than 5 members will be expected to have three female members. Supporters of the bill Democratic Sen. Connie Leyva of Chino said "We know that when boards are diverse and women's voices are heard, it's better for the whole workforce" and Sen. Hannah-Beth Jackson of Santa Barbara said "Yet another glass ceiling is shattered, and women will finally have a seat at the table in corporate boardrooms." In an ideal world, everyone wants company leadership to evaluate talent from all backgrounds of race and gender to select the best candidate, but because company's fail to give adequate attention to minority groups like Asian Americans and Women, people have to be watched over by government such as California. Violations consist of $300,000 for every occurence of not fulfilling the women board quota. Although the new law calls for improving gender diversity on public company boards, the legislation has drawn strong objections that employing quotas for women in board positions is poor public policy and unlawful with CAA Ambulance Association spokesman Chris Micheli saying "Gender is an important aspect of board diversity, but the state should not elevate this element over all other aspects of diversity."

The takeaway from women activists in the boardroom is for company leadership to promote diversity fairly without the need for States to intervene. Make diversity a part of your company culture - fairly considering Asian Americans for executive positions.

COMPANIES WITH ASIAN DISCRIMINATION

There are many instances where companies engage in racist actions from marketing campaigns, customer service, or employee interactions.

In 2017, United Airlines dragged David Dao, a 69-year-old Vietnamese Kentucky Doctor, forcibly off a United Airlines plane when he refused to give up his seat on the overbooked flight from Chicago O'Hare to Louisville, Kentucky when no one took the $800 offer to give up their seat. David Dao refused because he had patients to see the next day. Facebook videos went viral of David Dao being dragged off the plane unconscious dripping in blood from officers slamming his face into an armrest. Critics say David was targeted since he was an Asian American who would quietly accept being bumped. This PR crisis incident shocked many airlines to stop overbooking. To avoid public court hearings that would have humiliated the company since David Dao suffered a broken nose, a concussion, and broken teeth, United Airlines settled out of court with David Dao for $140 million.

In 2018, Dolce & Gabbana (D&G) posted a racist advertisement where a Chinese women struggles to eat pizza, spaghetti, and a cannoli with chopsticks. D&G first strike against Asians was slightly forgiven last year when the brand presented China as a third-world country where models surrounded themselves with poor Chinese people in underdeveloped parts of China. D&G's third strike was when D&G Founder Stefano Gabbana told Reuters about who will inherit his fortune "Once we will be dead, we will be dead. I don't want a Japanese designer to design for Dolce & Gabbana." Rightfully so, China, which accounts for more than 30% of D&G's sales, punished the brand with Tmall, JD.com, and Secoo all dropping D&G from their stores with many brands following suit. Chinese celebrities and key opinion leaders, who are critical to reaching Chinese customers, have also distanced themselves from the brand by publicly shaming D&G on Twitter and Weibo social media platforms. The severity of the meltdown was so large that D&G was forced to cancel their fashion show in Shanghai that was supposed to have 1,400 celebrities and influencers in attendance. Reuters reports that D&G lost as much as $500 million (33% of annual revenue) in revenue as a result of their racist mistake.

In 2004, Nike made a 90-second ad that attempted to fuse "Kill-Bill" concepts with basketball super powers showing LeBron James running laps around a bearded kung fu master resembling the one in "Kill Bill" movie and showing LeBron defeating two women wearing traditional Chinese attire and a pair of dragons. Upset with Nike disrespecting Chinese symbols, Chinese consumers voiced their disgust saying "This ad shows Chinese characters losing again and again. It makes our country look helpless against America." Chinese State Government officials said "Nike had violated the condition that all advertisements in China should uphold national dignity." Not wanting to lose sales from the lucrative Chinese market, Nike pulled the racist ad saying "We had no intention of hurting the emotions of Chinese consumers."

In 2002, Abercrombie and Fitch (A&F) pulled back racist shirts from all 311 shops in the United States that showed 2 men with slanted eyes in conical hats working for company "Wong Brothers Laundry Service" speaking broken English by saying "Two Wongs Can Make It White" that was meant to poke fun at "Two Wrongs Can Make It Right." The Organization of Chinese Americans said "We are outraged that the shirts would display degrading stereotypical Asian images and word plays solely for a corporation's profit." More than 100 Asian-Americans protested outside stores in San Francisco demanding that A&F issue a public apology in four major newspapers, increase philanthropic investment in the Asian community, and employment of consultants to ensure A&F handles Asian issues more sensitively going forward. San Francisco's Chinatown Community Development Center Program Director Norman Fong said "This is really blatant. It is just like the 1800s." Asian Pacific Islander Legal Outreach lawyer Ivy Lee says "It's unacceptable for them to smear and continue to perpetuate racist stereotypes of Asian-Americans. They wouldn't do the same for any other ethnic groups."

In 2018, Drybar, a nationwide salon chain which specializes in blow outs, had an employee who wrote "Chinky eyes" on Briana Tae's receipt at the Murray Hill location in New York City. Briana described the incident saying "When I confronted the front desk girl regarding this, she could not understand why it was an issue and why it was highly inappropriate to write such a description. I'm quite disgusted by this experience, especially the night before a day of celebration for all my accomplishments in nursing school." Drybar founder Alli Webb apologized saying "There was recently an unacceptable issue in one of our shops where a stylist described a client in a completely inappropriate way. We sincerely apologize for the hurt this has caused. We do not tolerate racism. The employee was immediately terminated, and we are committed to working harder on improving our training to ensure this does not happen again."

In 2016, Glamour Brasil made an Instagram post with team members slanting their eyes and bowing while on a trip to Japan. Glamour Brasil issued an apology saying "We apologize to the Asian community and every follower who has been offended by the publication in our Instagram account."

At service businesses, employees used racial slurs to describe customers such as at CVS in 2013 when a cashier labelled Hyun Lee's receipt as "Ching Chong Lee" where Hyun is seeking $1 million due to emotional distress, at Chick-fil-A where two Asian American UC Berkeley students received receipts of "ching & chong," at Taco Bell in 2018 when a cashier wrote "Steve Chink" ("chink" is a racist term) on student In Young Lee's receipt, and at Papa Johns where a cashier labelled Laura Cheifetz's pizza box as "ching-ching."

HOLLYWOOD ASIAN WHITEWASHING

In 2017, "Wonder Woman" Gal Gadot paved the way for aspiring women to become leading superhero stars in Hollywood typically dominated by male characters. In 2018, "Black Panther's" all-black cast paved the way for African-Americans to star in blockbuster films. Since Bruce Lee's death, Asian Americans still don't have a consistent talent pipeline of Asian Americans that are featured in top box office movies who are top earners in Hollywood consistently like Sofia Vergara, Dwayne Johnson, Kaley Cuoco, Denzel Washington, Scarlett Johansson, Tom Cruise, Angelina Jolie, George Clooney, Jennifer Lawrence, Robert Downey Jr, Gal Gadot, Will Smith, and many more.

An example of Asian Americans being treated unfairly by Hollywood producers is when Asian American "Hawaii Five-O" co-stars Grace Park and Daniel Dae Kim both left the show after producers refused to pay them as much as their fellow cast members. Daniel Dae Kim spoke out about his departure from the cast saying that he wanted to "maintain a steadfast sense of his self worth." Hollywood continues to underpay Asian Americans.

Don't even talk about getting highly paid like Dwayne Johnson or Scarlett Johansson, Asian Americans don't even get considered for cast auditions because of their last names as producers place stereotypes on Asians as people who have broken English accents and are physically weak. Marvel's

"Agents of Shield" star Chloe Bennet knows how hard it can be as an Asian-American actor in Hollywood with her last name "Wang." To overcome her last name stereotype for casting, Chloe changed her last name to Bennet and says "Oh, the first audition I went on after I changed my name, I got booked so that's a pretty clear little snippet of how Hollywood works...Hollywood is racist and wouldn't cast me with a last name that made them uncomfortable."

Chloe is also a critic of the constant whitewashing in Hollywood. Whitewashing is when characters originally written for Asian Americans have been given to white actors and actresses to portray in films. This is a shame. If Asian American kids grow up seeing Asian Americans being portrayed one way, they will shape their consciousness around that stereotype such as weak, shy, nerdy, unattractive, a coolie, the "butt of a joke," etc. For example, Jimmy Yang is portrayed in "Silicon Valley" as an Asian American who's nerdy, unattractive, weak, shy, and speaks broken English. Ken Jeong in the "Hangover" is portrayed as someone who speaks broken English and is weak. In "Full Metal Jacket" based on the Vietnam War, women prostitutes approach American soldiers for sex saying "Me love you long time...me sucky sucky...five dollar" which is degrading to Asian women who are approached by men like this in real life. Ryan Gosling in "The Big Short" movie makes fun of his Asian assistant saying "I trust this Asian's math as he won a math competition in China and doesn't even speak English!" - yet playing to the stereotype that Asians are nerdy, submissive, and speak broken English. Whitewashing is upsetting to the Asian American community when white characters play historically characters portrayed by Asian Americans such as Scarlett Johansson in "Ghost in the Shell," Matt Damon in "The Great Wall" with an Asian hair bun, Mickey Rooney in "Breakfast at Tiffany's," Tilda Swinton in "Doctor Strange," and Justin Chatwin in "Dragon Ball Z."

Once Hollywood begins to consistently cast Asian Americans in lead roles similar to Dwayne Johnson and Scarlett Johansson's of the world without whitewashing, Asian Americans will be more confident about succeeding in life as potential actors, actresses, and professionals.

Chloe Bennet applauded white actor Ed Skrein when he announced stepping down from a role in the "Hellboy" movie because he felt he would be "whitewashing" a character of Asian descent. Chloe told Ed "There is no way this decision came lightly on your part, so thank you for your bravery and genuinely impactful step forward. I hope this inspires other actors and film producers to not whitewash Asian characters."

One of the most controversial moments in Broadway history occurred in 1991 with the whitewashed role of the Engineer in "Miss Saigon" play. Powerful British producer Cameron Mackintosh was importing "Miss Saigon," a play with the most advance sales in Broadway history, from Britain to the US insisting that well-known white actor Jonathan Pryce play the role of the Engineer who is supposed to be French-Vietnamese. To look Asian, Jonathan Pryce wore prosthetics to alter the shape of his eyes and yellow makeup to make the color of his skin look Asian. This infuriated the Asian community. Anti-fans and Asian Americans viewed this whitewashing as racist leading to the rise of protest groups like "Don't Buy Miss Saigon" who organizes protests around musical performances. Until recently, "Miss Saigon" has only cast actors of Asian heritage to play the Engineer role. This is the type of corrective action that Hollywood needs to take in avoiding future whitewashing of Asian characters.

Sadly when Asian actors and actresses start getting more visible roles, they get bullied. Kelly Marie Tran, who played Rose Tico in "Star Wars: The Last Jedi," left Instagram as she was harassed on Tico's Wookieepedia page calling Kelly "Ching Chong Wing Tong" and listing Kelly's home as "Ching Chong China." Imagine if you were in Kelly's shoes, how would you feel?

HGTV star Joanna Gaines while in high school used to hide in the bathroom during lunch after being bullied for being Asian saying "My fear and my insecurities just took over and I felt like I'd rather sit in the stall than get rejected." Instead of seeking revenge, Joanna tells her five children to "look for that kid on the playground who's not playing with anybody and introduce yourself... look for the kid in the lunchroom who isn't sitting by anybody and be their friend." Heart broken in high school, Joanna trains her children to welcome kids who may feel bullied or left out as it can take a toll on their mental health.

In terms of non-Asian actors bullying Asian Americans, Mark Wahlberg is most famous when in April 1988 for assaulting a Vietnamese man by hitting him in the head with a large wooden stick until he was knocked unconscious while calling him a "Vietnam f**king shit." Mark was not done as he attacked a second Vietnamese man named Hoa "Johnny" Trinh by punching him in the eye while calling Johnny a "slant-eyed gook" - resulting in Johnny having one blind eye. For these crimes, Wahlberg served 45 days in jail and stained with a permanent felony record. As a popular actor who is opening many businesses, Mark should help educate his fans on treating the Asian community with respect or people will use his violent racism against him as Mark does not exhibit the qualities of a well-behaved human being.

Further damaging to the Vietnamese community occurred in 2018 when "Archer" voice actor Harry Jon Benjamin sent a racist tweet on Twitter saying "Quick idea for the name of a tea shop - 'ooh me so horny, me love you oolong time tea shop." After receiving backlash from the media, Harry quickly apologized saying "Sorry I offended many...The fact that it was a famous line in "Full Metal Jacket" movie does not give me license to stereotype Vietnamese people and Asian Americans in general. I'm sorry." Owning up is one thing and we just hope actors like Harry never again make racist comments that continue to hold back the Asian American community from thriving in Hollywood and life.

SINGERS MOCK ASIAN CULTURE

In the United States, there are no superstar role model singers of Asian descent who Caucasians and African Americans can look up to like Taylor Swift, Jay Z, Beyonce, Diddy, Katy Perry, The Weeknd, Drake, Pink, Kendrick Lamar, Ed Sheeran, Cardi B, Garth Brooks, Calvin Harris, Lady Gaga, Jimmy Buffett, and Luke Bryan. Instead, Asian Americans are the punchline of famous singers referenced in racial slurs. Nicki Minaj in her song "Chun Li," who is a female Asian character in the "Street Fighter" game, started the #ChunLiChallenge for followers to record themselves singing Nicki's song which led Asian American critics calling Nicki out for perpetuating racist Asian American stereotypes through cultural appropriation. Teen Vogue op-ed writer David Yi says the lyrics in Nicki's song including "I went and copped the chopsticks / put it in my bun just to pop sh*t" raises a red flag how cultural identities are reduced to gimmicks. What Nicki did per David is equivalent to "Chopsticks are eating utensils so it's about as appropriate as sticking forks in your hair which is considered extremely disrespectful, particularly in Japanese culture where it signifies death."

At the 2017 VMAs, Kendrick Lamar appropriated Asian culture where he surrounded himself with a handful of dancers dressed as ninjas doing various martial arts and later climbing a wall of fire..

Lil Pump in "Butterfly Doors" song sings "Smoking on dope, they call me Yao Ming cause my eye real low" while pulling his eyelids in a common gesture mocking Asians.

Love can get testy especially between two races such as when Rihanna made racist comments towards her ex-boyfriend Chris Brown's half Vietnamese girlfriend Karrueche Tran by tweeting a photo of a bag of rice cakes with the caption "Ima make u my b****" which was perceived as being a racial insult at Tran.

Wiz Khalifa in the song "Hot Now" contained the lyrics "Smoke got my eyes looking Korean" enraged the Asian American community and Wiz refuses to apologize.

In 2009, Miley Cyrus took a pictures with friends slanting their eyes which sets a poor example for her young fans causing the Asian advocate group OCA saying "the picture falls within a long and unfortunate history of people mocking and denigrating individuals of Asian descent." Miley apologized for her insensitivity of the Asian community.

The Chainsmokers mocked China saying "we wouldn't bring a dog to China as Chinese people eat dogs." To appease their Asian friends in China, The Chainsmokers said "We would never intentionally do anything to upset our fans and we apologize if it offended anyone."

TV SHAMES ASIAN BROKEN ENGLISH

In TV, Asian Americans don't have role models such as Oprah Winfrey, Ellen DeGeneres, Conan O'Brien, Jimmy Fallon, Jimmy Kimmel, or Stephen Colbert. Instead, notable TV personalities bring down the Asian community thru racist comments towards Asians as a punch line.

In 2016 Fox News' Jesse Watters interviewed Asian Americans who spoke broken English in New York City's Chinatown. The five-minute video began with an instrumental version of the "Kung Fu Fighting" song mixed with scenes of Jesse getting a foot massage and playing with nunchucks. Offended, elected officials and activists protested outside Fox News' headquarters. New York City Mayor Bill de Blasio said "The vile, racist behavior of Fox's Jesse Watters in Chinatown has no place in our city." New York City Councilman Peter Koo said "Passing off this blatantly racist television segment as 'gentle fun' not only validates racist stereotypes, it encourages them. The entire segment smacks of willful ignorance by buying into the perpetual foreigner syndrome." Renee Tajima-Peña, a professor of Asian-American studies at UCLA, says "That kind of duality of the perception of Asians has been there since time...We are either perpetual foreigners or we are the favored model minority...We are a threat or we are docile." Very disappointing to see professionals as Jesse spread hateful messages to a large audience.

Rosie O'Donnell mocked Chinese on "The View" saying "you can imagine in China it's like 'Ching chong. Danny DeVito, ching chong.'" After being educated on Asian culture, Rosie said "To say ching chong to someone is very offensive, and some Asian people have told me it's as bad as the n-word...But I'm also gonna give you a fair warning that there's a good chance I'll do something like that again, probably in the next week -- not on purpose. Only 'cause it's how my brain works." Disgusted, Karen Lincoln Michel, president of Unity Journalists of Color Inc says "I think by allowing Rosie O'Donnell's cheap jabs at Chinese Americans to go unchecked, the network is essentially condoning racial and ethnic slurs." When TV show hosts make racist remarks such as Rosie did towards the Asian community, she must be punished or will continue to hurt the Asian community with her insensitive remarks.

Some TV host such as Nick Cannon are honest about being racist when Nick says "All the racists in here make some noise. I'm racist too...If I meet somebody from India, I assume their house smell like curry. My Asian friends, I don't let them walk my dog because they might wok my dog! If I see a middle-aged white man in some sweatpants by a school, pedophile!" This was shocking to hear and we can only hope someone educates Nick about global culture as these words could cause his followers to become racist towards Indians, Asians, and White Men.

COMEDIANS EMASCULATE ASIAN MEN

Asian Americans don't have comedian role models such as Kevin Hart or Jerry Sienfeld at the top of the profession. Instead Asian Americans are the butt of the joke such as at the 2016 Oscars when Chris Rock portrayed three common Asian American stereotypes when he brought 3 Asian boys on stage dressed as accountants: the model minority student who is a math genius, the foreign child laborer who assembles tech gadgets for pennies, and the silent obedient immigrant whom we can project whatever identity we please because they won't fight back. At the Oscars, Chris Rock introduced the three Asian boys as "Ming Zhu, Bao Ling, and David Moskowitz" saying they are "the most dedicated, accurate, and hard-working accountants at PricewaterhouseCoopers...If anybody is upset about that joke, just tweet about it on your phone that was also made by these kids."

Recognizing Chris Rock's racist mistake, the Academy spokesperson issued the statement, "The Academy regrets that any aspect of the Oscar telecast was offensive. We are committed to doing our best to ensure that material in future shows be more culturally sensitive." Disgusted, "Crazy Rich Asians" star Constance Wu said "To parade little kids on stage with no speaking lines merely to be the butt of a racist joke is reductive and gross. Antithesis of progress."

Amy Schumer famous for publicly admitting she's had sex with 28 different men hurt the Asian community by emasculating Asian men saying "I think my parents would be mad if I brought home an Asian guy. They would be like 'I don't understand. Do you really want to f**k this guy?'"

In 2018 disgraced comedian Louis C.K., who is a #metoo offender for masturbating naked in front of 5 women without their consent, emasculated Asian men in his leaked comedy stand-up saying "You know why Asian guys have small dicks....Because they're women. They're not dudes. They're all women. All Asians are women. And they have big clits, really big clits, and when they have sex they just stick their clits in each other's pussies and then they procreate using math." Asian Americans are growing tired of continuous mockery of Asian men with Washington Post's Gene Park saying "Ok Louis CK's Asian man jokes puts him at Amy Schumer levels of unfunny (she also made similar, tired jokes). Forget social commentary, this is just sad" and New York Magazine's E. Alex Jung saying "The fact that Louis CK's anti-asian jokes weren't originally reported speaks volumes to how casually americans still treat anti-asian racism. same with chappelle. same with tiffany haddish."

On "The Tonight Show With Jay Leno" in 2007, Chelsea Handler made a racist remark to Angelina Jolie's adopted son Pax saying "Pax probably doesn't even know he's Asian yet. He certainly doesn't know he's going to be a horrible driver. Or that he's going to be amazing at doing nails. He has no idea!" Yet again, perpetuating Asian stereotypes.

In 2001 during Conan O'Brien's show, Sarah Silverman made a racist remark when she advised her friend on avoiding jury duty by writing a racial slur on the selection form such as "I hate chinks" or "I love chinks." Sarah Silverman debated with Asian American activist Guy Aoki about using the word "chink" on Bill Maher's "Politically Incorrect" show with no apology from Sarah.

In 2017, Steve Harvey mocked self-help book titled "How to Date a White Woman: A Practical Guide for Asian Men," saying "neither Black nor white women desire Asian men...That's one page...You like Asian men?...I don't even like Chinese food...I don't eat what I can't pronounce." The crowd uncomfortably laughed along with Steve, but the Asian community was furious. In an open letter to The New York Times, "Fresh Off the Boat" author Eddie Huang said "Harvey perpetuates the stereotype that women don't want Asian men...Harvey speaks openly about issues facing the black community. Unfortunately for his own personal profit, he's willing to perpetuate the emasculation of Asian men." Rarely apologizing, Steve says "I offer the humblest apology for offending anyone, particularly those in the Asian community. It was not my intention and the humor was not meant with any malice or disrespect whatsoever." Too many instances of racism towards Asian American. High profile comedians like Steve must know better.

FASHION MODELS BELITTLE ASIAN WOMEN

There are not many Asians featured as Victoria's Secret angels. Asian Americans don't have role models of Asian descent to look up to like non-Asians have with Gisele Bundchen, Adriana Lima, Miranda Kerr, Kendall Jenner, Karlie Kloss, Heidi Klum, Kate Moss, Bella Hadid, and Gigi Hadid. Asian Americans has only one success so far when Liu Wen proved that Asian models could be part of the Victoria Secret's Fashion Show in 2009 and made history in 2017 when Liu became the first Asian model to appear on the cover of "American Vogue."

In the 2018 Miss Universe competition, Miss USA Sarah Rose Summers mocked "Top 5 finisher" Miss Vietnam H'Hen Niê for speaking broken English. This led to Sarah Rose Summers being shamed as the "Ambassador of Bullying."

At the 2017 Shanghai Fashion show, Gigi Hadid was labeled a racist in China after an Instagram video surfaced of Gigi and her friends taking a photo with slanted eye gesture. As punishment, Gigi and her friends in the video were denied visas into China for the Shanghai Fashion show for their racist gestures to the Asian community.

NFL PLAYERS VIEW ASIANS AS WEAK

Few Asian Americans have made the NFL. There has yet to be a pipeline of Asian American stars like non-Asians have with Tom Brady, Peyton Manning, Drew Brees, Aaron Rodgers, Cam Newton, Jimmy Garoppolo, Michael Vick, Khalil Mack, Aaron Donald, Adrian Peterson, Todd Gurley, Von Miller, Mike Evans, Calvin Johnson, Julio Jones, Antonio Brown, and Odell Beckham Jr.

Dat Nguyen, a Vietnamese American, played for the Dallas Cowboys from 1999-2005. With no Asian American role model, Walter Payton was Dat's idol, inspiring Dat to become an All-American linebacker at Texas A&M. At the 2017 College Football Hall of Fame Dat said "I was in a unique position just because I was Asian, and Texas A&M had never seen an Asian linebacker play the position...I carry this as a chip on my shoulders...My parents left Vietnam in the fall of Saigon in 1975...when I wore the name on the back of my shoulder pads I was representing not just my community and my family at Texas A&M but also the country of Vietnam."

In 2010 Ed Wang, a left tackle from Virginia Tech, became the first Chinese American football player drafted in the NFL Draft. Wang has dealt with racism on the field as he was usually the only Asian on his football and basketball teams. By overcoming the racism in making it to the NFL, Wang hopes that his ability to get drafted will inspire other Asian Americans to play football.

It is disappointing when non-Asian players make racist remarks to the Asian community or Asian staff. Richie Incognito did that when he, Jerry and Pouncey made racial slurs at the Assistant Trainer calling him as a "Jap," "Chinaman," "chink," "dirty communist," and a "North Korean." All three spoke to the Assistant Trainer of Japanese descent in a broken English accent asking for "rubby rubby sucky sucky" in reference to the "Full Metal Jacket" movie, called his mother a "rub and tug masseuse," and saying that they had had sex with his girlfriend.

New England Patriots star Rob Gronkowski in a video captured by TMZ referred to an Asian man in the crowd at a party as "Leslie Chow," the Ken Jeong character in "Hangover" movie saying "They told me he could only cook fried rice." Rob apologized for his insensitive comments towards the Asian community.

In 2018, Christian Fauria a WEEI radio host was suspended five days by WEEI after impersonating Tom Brady's agent Don Yee with a stereotypical Asian accent. Yee, a Chinese-American born in California speaks with no accent. To encourage Christian to learn about the Asian culture, Don Yee invited Christian to participate in an Asian American Journalists Association (AAJA) panel about racial ignorance toward Asians in the media. After the panel Christian said "Being called a racist is the worst thing in the world. As a father of four children who are a quarter Japanese and Korean, I played them the radio clip mocking Agent Yee...One of my daughters ran off crying. They were very upset and I just explained to them that what I did was wrong."

BASEBALL PLAYERS THINK ASIANS ARE TWINS

Few Asian Americans have made the MLB. Asian Americans don't have superstar role models like David Ortiz, Manny Ramirez, Derek Jeter, Alex Rodriguez, Clayton Kershaw, Mike Trout, Giancarlo Stanton, Albert Pujols, David Price, Max Scherzer, Felix Hernandez, Stephen Strasburg, Miguel Cabrera, Aaron Judge, Mookie Betts, and Bryce Harper to look up to.

In 2018, the Los Angeles Angels hosted the Seattle Mariners with Japanese superstars Shohei Ohtani and Ichiro Suzuki playing in the same ballpark. MLB Twitter posted a photo of Shohei shaking hands with Ichiro with the troubling caption "Spiderman pointmeme" hinting that all Asians look alike. In response, fans critiqued MLB for being racist with lack of social awareness. One critic said "What's worse is that MLB deleted the tweet, haven't apologized and are pretending that the racist post never happened."

In 2017, Boston Red Sox broadcaster Jerry Remy apologized after suggesting on-field translators should be illegal during a Boston-New York Yankees game saying "pitchers like Japanese-born Yankees star Masahiro Tanaka should learn baseball language without the need for on-field translators." In response to racist remarks made by Jerry, NESN television network says "NESN does not agree with any such views expressed by Jerry Remy and we know from talking to Jerry that he regrets making them and the network sincerely apologizes to anyone who was offended by Jerry's comments" and Jerry apologized saying "I'd like to apologize to my colleagues at NESN, to the Boston Red Sox but most importantly to the fans who were offended by my comments. I sincerely hope you accept my apologies."

During the 2017 Houston Astros World Series Championship run, Houston Astros Cuban-native Yuli Gurriel was banned five games for a racist gesture by pulling his eyes back after he homered off Los Angeles Dodgers Japanese pitcher Yu Darvish. Upset, Yu Darvish says "Yuli was disrespectful...There should be punishment levied as a learning lesson for making insensitive racist remarks." The Houston Astros donated the $322,581 Yuli lost over five games to a charity supporting diversity efforts. This punishment was not enough per Asian American member saying "Rob's failure to punish Yuli during the World Series says baseball has a long way to go in protecting players from racism."

In 2014, New York Mets pitching coach Dan Warthen used a racial slur towards Daisuke Matsuzaka's Japanese American interpreter. In response to the racist remarks Dan says "I'm sorry I called you a Chinaman. I apologize for the thoughtless remarks that I made in the clubhouse. They were a poor attempt at humor but were wrong and inappropriate in any setting and I am very sorry" and General Manager Sandy Alderson said "On behalf of the entire organization, I apologize for the insensitive remarks made by pitching coach Dan Warthen. The remarks were offensive and inappropriate and the organization is very sorry."

In 2018, San Francisco Giants Pitcher Derek Holland brought out the Giants' Japanese massage therapist Haro Ogawa as a punch line by making Haro stand silently near Holland for Holland to make a series of lame jokes in a Japanese accent while mockingly bowing to Haro after each joke. In response to Holland's racist behavior, Giants spokesperson Matt Chisholm says "The Giants organization does not condone that type of behavior in any way. We spoke to Derek regarding his interview yesterday and he completely understands the severity of the situation and he apologizes if it offended anyone" and Derek says "I apologize for what I've done. I don't want to offend anybody. I apologize for doing that. I want to be held accountable."

NBA PLAYERS SAY ASIANS ARE WEAK

Few Asian Americans have made the NBA with no Asian American role models such as African Americans have with Michael Jordan, LeBron James, Kobe Bryant, Shaquille O'Neal, Carmelo Anthony, Stephen Curry, Kevin Durant, Tim Duncan, Joel Embiid, Anthony Davis, Russell Westbrook, Chris Paul, James Harden, and Kevin Garnett. Instead, the occasional Asian basketball players face racial discrimination as happened in 2003 when Los Angeles Lakers legend Shaquille O'Neal told a Chinese reporter to tell Houston Rockets Chinese basketball player Yao Ming "Tell Yao Ming Ching-chong-yang-wah-ah-so." Shaq says this before meeting Yao for the first time since Yao Ming was drafted #1 overall in the 2002 NBA Draft - posing as the first real threat to Shaq's dominance at the center position. In response, the Organization of Chinese Americans (OCA) held a news conference to condemn Shaq's remarks prior to Houston's game against the Los Angeles Lakers which is when Shaq and Yao met on the court for the first time as rival NBA centers. In a statement to the NBA, the OCA said "Shaq's derogatory and racial taunt ching-chong-yang-wah-ah-soh aimed at Yao was racially offensive and particularly harmful to the millions of Asian Americans who aspire to become great basketball players like Yao Ming in a sport dominated by non-Asians." Shaq did not apologize further cementing the racism double standard that its unacceptable for people to make racist comments towards

African Americans but is meant to be a joke when African Americans make racist jokes to Asians.

When Yao Ming retired in 2011, Asian Americans didn't have a role model to look up to until New York Knicks Jeremy Lin dazzled for two weeks in February 2012 with fans calling the moment "Linsanity." Immediately, Jeremy experienced racism in a sport dominated by non-Asians when Fox Sports columnist Jason Whitlock tweeted "Some lucky lady in NYC is gonna feel a couple of inches of pain tonight." This is disgusting as someone with NBA-level talent like Jeremy still faces harassment and bullying because of his appearance and background. Jeremy recalls the racism experienced when he played basketball at Harvard University especially against Yale where opposing fans heckled "Hey! Can you even see the scoreboard with those eyes?" Even when Asian players do well, they still experience racism.

In 2008 at the Beijing Olympics, Spain's Pau Gasol apologised on behalf of his team when 15 players pulled back their eyes in a photo for team sponsor Seur saying "If anyone feels offended, we totally apologise for it."

In 2001, Sacramento Kings Jason Williams responded to NBA fan Michael Ching who told Jason "to get used to sitting on the bench" with racist remarks saying "I'll shoot all you slant-eyed Asian mother———. Do you remember the Vietnam War? I'll shoot you like that." Williams was fined $15,000, which is a slap on the wrist considering his $10 million-plus salary. The NBA has to do more in ensuring players and fans of all ethnicities can comfortably enjoy the game of basketball without experiencing racism.

Historically in 1947, the year Jackie Robinson broke MLB baseball's color barrier, 5-foot-7 inch Japanese-American point guard Wat Misaka from Utah was drafted by the New York Knicks as the first non-White player drafted into the NBA. This was an extremely difficult time for an Asian athlete as 1947 was just 1 year after the end of internment camps in Western America where 120,000 Japanese Americans were jailed during World War II.

In addition to Asian Americans experiencing racism, Jewish people do as well and it was sad to see NBA Superstar LeBron James make an Instagram post saying "need to get that Jewish money." With over 46 million Instagram followers, LeBron James quickly apologized but this is not enough as the NBA has to ensure all teams teach their players and communities to respect people from all walks of life. We don't want to run into a situation such as the 2018 Pittsburgh Synagogue Shooting where an anti-semitic gunman killed 11 Jewish people.

NHL HOCKEY HAS 0 ASIAN STARS

Few Asian Americans play in the NHL with no role models like Caucasian players have with Wayne Gretzky, Sidney Crosby, Patrick Kane, Evgeni Malkin, Steven Stamkos, Zach Parise, Ryan Suter, and Alex Ovechkin.

Less than a year after Jackie Robinson shattered the baseball color line, Larry Kwong broke the barrier in hockey on March 13, 1948 when he made his NHL debut with the New York Rangers. Kwong experienced racism growing up in Vernon where as a young adult, he was offered a job as a hotel bellboy while his teammates were given well-paid jobs at the local smelter. Kwong says "I made the team, but they wouldn't give me a job because I was Chinese."

Larry Woo, father of Vancouver Canucks hockey player Jett Woo, recalls that people would bring chopsticks to games he played in as a teenager in Canada's Western Hockey League to mock him for being Asian with racist gestures and racial slurs. Fortunately Larry's son Jett Woo, who was drafted in the second round of the 2018 National Hockey League (NHL) draft by the Vancouver Canucks, hasn't experienced racism like his parents did. Larry says the backstory of Jett's name is a tribute to Jet Li because "Jet Li was coming to Winnipeg and my parents were going to be his host family but he decided to go to Hollywood...Like Bruce and Jet kicked down doors in Hollywood, I hope Jett Woo can be a trailblazer in the NHL."

SOCCER DOESN'T SCOUT ASIANS

Few Asian Americans succeed at the highest level of soccer in Europe and South America like Lionel Messi, Cristiano Ronaldo, Neymar, Gareth Bale, Paul Pogba, Luis Suarez, Kylian Mbappe, James Rodriguez, Zlatan Ibrahimovic, Alexis Sanchez, Mesut Ozil, and Kevin De Bruyne.

Being able to play for the 20 English Premier League teams in the United Kingdom is the goal for many soccer players with teams like Manchester City, Manchester United, Newcastle United, Liverpool, Everton, Arsenal, Chelsea, Leicester City, Tottenham Hotspur, and other elite teams. In 2018 at the British Sociological Association's annual conference in Newcastle, soccer scouts admitted they ignore Asian players because they thought Asian players were only interested in non-contact sports such as cricket. Dr. Dan Kilvington Leeds Beckett University told the conference that only 12 out of over 3,700 (.32%) professional players in the United Kingdom are of Asian ethnicity even though British Asians account for 5 percent of the general population and that Asians participate more in amateur football than Caucasians. Dr. Kilvington says the lack of Asian players in the English Premier League is due to stereotype among scouts that Asians are weak, lack of Asian coaches at grassroots level, and absence of Asian role models for players – there was only one Asian football coach out of 522 senior coaches in England.

In 2013, Shinji Kagawa of Borussia Dortmund became the first Asian player to score a hat-trick in the English Premier League. However in 2017, anti-racism group Kick It Out called on Manchester United to punish any fans involved in a racially offensive video singing "His name is Shinji, Shinji, Shinji! His grandad bombed Pearl Harbour, Pearl Harbour, Pearl Harbour!"

South Korea National Team Captain Son Heung-min is one of the most high-profile Asian players in Europe playing for the Tottenham Hotspur. He's faced racism his entire life especially in 2018 during a match against West Ham when a West Ham fan screamed "f**king chink." With Son as a role model star for Asian fans, Asian fans experience racism just for enjoying a game such as in 2018 when fans at Wembley used racist stereotypes towards an Asian fan behind them saying "Son…has he got his egg fried rice. Chicken chow mein?" In response, Tottenham banned the racist fans from attending future matches saying "Any kind of racist, discriminatory or anti-social behaviour will not be tolerated by Tottenham. We have a strict, zero tolerance attitude in this regard and shall take action against anyone behaving or using language that is abusive, offensive or obscene." Another incident of racism occurred in 2018 when Chilean midfielder Diego Valdes pulled his eyes back in a photo with a South Korean fan. Valdes apologized saying "In relation to the photograph that has appeared on social media, it was never my intention to offend and I offer my apologies to anyone that could have been offended" whereas Chilean Coach Reinaldo Rueda provided a disgraceful response saying "This is a press conference to talk about soccer. I am not here to talk about things not related to soccer." As a leader, Coach Rueda should have addressed racism and punished Valdes right away. This response hints that Coach Rueda condones racism.

In 2018 when South Korea's win over Germany at the FIFA World Cup helped Mexico into the knockout stages, fans including NBC's Telemundo host James Tahhan in Mexico City rushed to the South Korean embassy to party while posting pictures of themselves pulling their eyes back, which is considered a racist gesture. James Tahhan apologised on Twitter saying "I made an inappropriate and insensitive gesture towards the Asian community. I want to apologise to anyone who was offended by it."

In 2017, Colombian National Team's Edwin Cardona apologized for his actions during the game against South Korea when Cardona pulled his eyes back. The Colombian Football Federation apologized for Cardona's actions to both the South Korean players as well as the country. Cardona's actions were condemned by the Korean media and captain Ki Sung-yeung saying "Racist behavior is unacceptable. Colombia is a team full of world-class players and it was disappointing to see this kind of thing." FIFA banned Cardona five games.

In 2017, Chelsea's Brazilian star Kenedy was sent home from China after his offensive Instagram video of an asleep security guard with the caption "Wake up China, You Idiot." Furious, The People's Daily newspaper said "China does not welcome a player like this, nor does China welcome a team like this. Kenedy's absurd comments are not only impolite but also uneducated. He has created an incident that has humiliated China, an incident that so many fans simply cannot tolerate." Kenedy's Chelsea attempted to save face from China with their statement "His behaviour does not represent the entire team. He has been disciplined. Everyone at Chelsea Football Club has the utmost respect and admiration for China and loves our Chinese fans. It is because of this that the negative impact we have seen over the last two days has left us shocked and saddened. We have listened carefully to the criticism and will use the lessons learnt over the last two days to improve our processes in future."

In 2015, English Premier League's top player Jamie Vardy of Leicester City regrets his terrible mistake in racially abusing an Asian man in a casino for calling him a "Jap." Jamie thought his career was over saying "Most convictions get wiped after a period of time. But there's no way of erasing what happened in July 2015. The word 'racist' is a permanent stain against my name. It's worse than a criminal record. It's on YouTube and Google when my kids type in their dad's name and it comes up 'Jamie Vardy racist.'"

GOLF DOESN'T HAVE ASIAN CHAMP

Asian Americans don't have golf role models like Caucasians do with Phil Mickelson, Annika Sorenstam, Rory McIllroy, Karrie Webb, Cristie Kerr, Jordan Spieth, Stacy Lewis, Dustin Johnson, Paula Creamer, Bubba Watson, and Beth Daniel.

Unfortunately Asian golfers encounter racism such as in 2003 when Australian Women's Golfer Jan Stephenson told Golf Magazine "Asians are killing women's golf. There should be quotas to limit the percentage of Asians on the LPGA Tour." This infuriated the Asian community including "A Magazine" publisher Jeff Yang who said "Somehow it's OK to suggest restrictions against Asians because we won't fight back and we are fundamentally more foreign." MSNBC conducted a poll asking "Is Jan Stephenson right that Asian players are hurting the LPGA Tour?" 50% of the 8,439 responses said yes which disappointed Jeff Yang who said "Does half of America think Latinos are hurting baseball? That African-Americans are hurting basketball? That Europeans are hurting hockey? Let's hope not. Because those groups, much like Koreans in the LPGA, are making their sports remarkably better. And still somehow, half of the MSNBC.com poll respondents think Asians are hurting women's golf."

TENNIS LACKS ASIAN STARS

Asian Americans don't have tennis role models like non-Asians do with Roger Federer, Rafael Nadal, Novak Djokovic, Serena Williams, Caroline Wozniacki, Venus Williams, Andy Murray, Maria Sharapova, Pete Sampras, Andre Agassi, and Sloane Stephens.

In 1989 Michael Chang made tennis history when he won the French Open at the age of 17 years, 110 days to become the youngest male player ever to win a Grand Slam title. As a rare Asian American tennis player at the top of the game, Michael said "I felt like there was added pressure. Obviously the Asian American community wants you to do well." Michael's victory over third-ranked Stefan Edberg in the French Open final inspired many Asian Americans to pick up tennis as they wanted "to be like Mike." Great players give back to the community and Michael did just that when Jeremy Lin entered the NBA as a potential Asian American star telling Jeremy "I had doubters who looked at me and figured I was too small, too passive, too unathletic. It was unfathomable for someone to utter 'Asian American' and 'professional athlete' in the same sentence" which inspired Jeremy to go on his "Linsanity" run in 2012 with the New York Knicks.

To help Asian tennis players overcome the "Asians are "soft" stereotype, China's two-time Grand Slam Singles Champion Li Na advised Asian tennis players Naomi Osaka, Kei Nishikori, Qiang Wang, Hyeon Chung, Saisai Zheng, Shuai Zhang, Yuichi Sugita, and Yafan Wang saying "modesty is a typical trait of Asian culture that holds players back so you have to be intense in showing the world you are great."

Even Asian tennis officials experience racism such as in 2017 when Brazilian Guilherme Clezar mockingly stretched his eyes after he successfully challenged a line judge's call during a match against Japan's Yuichi Sugita. With the Asian community angered, the International Tennis Federation (ITF) fined Clezar for unsportsmanlike conduct saying "Clezar issued a written apology. The ITF condemns all forms of offensive behaviour" and Clezar apologized saying "Even though I didn't mean any prejudice, I recognise the gesture doesn't ring true with the attitudes of respect, enthusiasm, solidarity, emotion and many other things that sport means to us and I want to express my regret and my most sincere apologies."

COLLEGES BULLY SMART & SHY ASIANS

Entrance to elite American universities should be based on merit as judged by college's admissions selection committee, but investigations in 2018 revealed that Ivy League colleges Harvard University, Yale University, Brown University, and Dartmouth College were biased against Asian American applicants as the universities used a "personal rating" score which includes subjective factors such as being nice and likable. Universities have complained that Asians score too high on standardized tests like the SAT and AP exams than all other races. Because merit is not 100% valued in admissions, the United States Department of Justice is investigating these universities saying "the DOJ takes seriously any potential violation of an individual's constitutional rights." The Asian American Coalition for Education is also a plaintiff in the lawsuit against Harvard University saying "the school's race-conscious admissions policy discriminates against Asian-Americans." Regarding discrimination, a Princeton study found that Asians needed to score 140 points higher on the SAT than whites for admission into the best colleges - a difference some have called "the Asian tax."

When Asians at elite universities work hard to achieve good grades for great careers, students experience racism such as in 2018 when Han Ju Seo was studying in the library at Washington University in St. Louis being yelled "Why are Asian students invading OUR campus study spaces" and replied back to her school community saying "Thanks for the reminder that no matter my citizenship, the years I've spent in America, and my proficiency in English, I'm always going to be a foreigner. No matter how much we excel in our careers, achieve incredible things, and work to the point of utter exhaustion we're still unwanted. Go ahead and love my culture, love my food, and love my music; call me when I'm welcome. I'm tired." In response to Han Ju Seo's depression, Washington University responded "These messages are inconsistent with the university's goal of creating an inclusive and diverse environment and are just one example of the broader bias and oppression that Asian and Asian American students experience."

In 2011 at UCLA, student Alexandra Wallace posted a YouTube video ranting about Asian students using cellphones in the library saying "OHH CHING CHONG TING TONG LING LONG... OHH." In response to the outrage for Alexandra's racist remarks, Alexandra responded saying "I have offended the UCLA community and the entire Asian culture. I am truly sorry for the hurtful words I said and the pain it caused to anyone who watched the video. Especially in the wake of the ongoing disaster in Japan, I would do anything to take back my insensitive words."

Many Asian Americans gain admission to elite universities solely thru academics whereas athletes have a lower test score minimum for admission. Although most college students don't play at the professional level, athletics provides students with camaraderie and fitness during college. The NCAA has a database to track the demographics of student-athletes in the United States and the statistics are troubling for Asian athletes. In college baseball, 318 of 34,980 (.9%) student-athletes were Asian. In college football, 386 of 73,057 (.53%) student-athletes were Asian. In college basketball, 107 of 18,712 (.57%) student-athletes were Asian. In college ice hockey, 28 of 4,197 (.67%) student-athletes were Asian. Similar to professional soccer, Asian college athletes are underrepresented due to lack of scouting.

College students with the highest grades (GPA) and campus experience (play a Division 1 sport) tend to get the best paid job offers in Wall Street finance jobs, Silicon Valley tech jobs, and graduate school admission. It's critical that university leadership ensure that all students achieve their grades thru merit instead of grade inflation such as UNC (Michael Jordan's college) did by helping 3,100 student-athletes over 18 years take fake paper classes in African American studies to stay eligible, Southern University in Louisiana where 541 students paid Deputy Registrar Cleo Carroll to award them higher grades ($500 per F to A grade and $200 per B to A grade) and fake diplomas ($1,600 for a fake official university transcript); Computer Science major students cheating at Harvard University, Stanford University, and Brown University for Silicon Valley jobs with Facebook and Google; Florida State University where two tutors provided online test answers to 61 athletes including 25 football players, and University of Minnesota tutors who wrote more than 400 papers for 20 players on the men's basketball team.

Mental health is extremely important as 1 in 5 college students consider suicide from stress per a survey conducted by Cindy Liu of Brigham and Women's Hospital's developmental risk and cultural disparities program.

Stressful events include academic pressures, career issues, love and relationships;,personal appearance, personal health problems, and sleep difficulties. Liu's team found that 3 out of 4 students in the 67,000 survey had experienced at least one stressful event in the previous year. For Asian and Asian American males, Dr. Henry Chung, the student health AVP at New York University (NYU) and executive director of the NYU Student Health Center, says "Asian-American/Asian students, especially males, are under unique pressures to meet high expectations of parents by succeeding in such traditional predetermined careers as medicine and engineering. Immigrant groups feel pressures due to sacrifices made by family members for their children's benefit." Regarding Asian women, California State University Fullerton Asian American Studies Professor Eliza Noh, who dedicated her life to study suicide issues among Asian women after her younger sister killed herself with a gun in 1990 as a college junior, says "the stereotype of model minority for Asian women is overwhelming. They fall in depression or commit suicide when they cannot meet the expectations from the family and the society."

Before 2018 when America took mental health seriously due to suicidal deaths by celebrities Kate Spade and Anthony Bourdain, colleges did not dedicate mental health resources for students especially at elite universities like Cornell University where 13 out of 21 (62%) on-campus suicides between 1996-2006 involved Asian Americans students, at MIT where 8 out of 19 (42%) on-campus suicides between 2000-2015 involved Asian American students, at Stanford University in 2007 when May Zhou committed suicide after overdosing on three bottles of Unisom sleeping pills while laying in the trunk of her car, at Harvard University in 2015 when Luke Tang committed suicide after people saved him from a suicide attempt earlier in the year, at Brown University in 2015 when Hyoun Ju Sohn committed suicide by jumping from the 12th floor of the science building, at Columbia University in 2018 when Kirk Wu hung himself in the student bathroom, at Yale University in 2016 when the daughter-in-law of CJ Group's Chairman Rae Na Lee committed suicide and in 2015 when Luchang Wang committed suicide by jumping off the San Francisco Golden Gate Bridge, at Princeton University in 2016 when Wonshik Shin committed suicide in his dorm room, and at California Institute of Technology where 3 Asian students committed suicide within three months in 2009.

At Boston University, social research professor Hyeouk Chris Hahm is conducting a study called Asian Women's Action for Resilience and Empowerment (AWARE) sponsored by the National Institutes of Health to study the mental health of second-generation Asian-American women because Asian-American women ages 18 to 24 have the nation's second-highest suicide rate (per NIH 2012 data) among women in this age group behind Native Americans. The NIH awarded Hahm's AWARE program a grant to create intervention programs. In 2016 at Wellesley College, a college where 22% of students are Asian, they became the first school in America to implement an intervention program saying "We believe that the whole student needs to be supported and that for students to understand themselves, they need to understand their own history, family structure, cultural background, as well as the gendered and racial structures that influence the way they see themselves and are seen by others."

SCHOOLS BULLY SHY ASIAN KIDS

1st generation Asian Americans like myself were raised by parents who sacrificed their lives in coming to America so their children can achieve the American Dream of a great career by demonstrating merit thru test scores and grades. In the land of opportunity, all children should be rewarded based on their merit not on their skin color or family's net worth.

In 2019, New York City Mayor Bill de Blasio proposed plans to reserve 20% of the 4,000 total seats for admission to the city's eight nationally-recognized high schools like Stuyvesant High School, the Bronx High School of Science, and Brooklyn Technical High School, for students from high poverty schools. Angered, Asian American parents of students at New York City's elite public schools have filed a federal lawsuit against Mayor Bill de Blasio discriminating against Asian-American children. Yi Fang Chen, who moved to the U.S. from China with her parents in 1996, said in a statement "We all have the American dream of equal opportunity. I was able to achieve what my parents came to this country for. But by using race preference to determine student enrollment at these excellent schools, it's like the Mayor is taking someone else's dream away." The plaintiffs in the lawsuit include Asian-American parents, the Asian American Coalition for Education, and the Chinese American Citizens Alliance of Greater New York Admission Test. President of the Stuyvesant alumni association Soo Kim furiously said "Correct me if I'm wrong, but they're saying these schools are too Asian. I don't understand how that's even legal." New York City Councilman Peter Koo says "The test is the most unbiased way to get into a school. It doesn't require a resume. It doesn't even require connections. The Mayor's son just graduated from Brooklyn Tech and got into Yale. Now he wants to stop this and build a barrier to Asian-Americans -- especially our children. These schools are especially important for our understanding of meritocracy, because many see admissions to those universities as the ultimate demonstration of merit."

America is regarded as one of the best countries in the World to obtain a college education. You don't want to see schools cheat children for financial gains such as the 178 teachers and principals from 44 City of Atlanta Georgia public schools did on the State Exams in 2009 - the biggest school cheating scandal in U.S. History. If you are a parent of a low-performing student or are a low-performing student, you should be motivated to improve your intellectual capabilities based on your merit not thru cheating.

Bullying is a big concern for Asian Americans. A 2017 survey found that Asian American teenagers suffered far more bullying at school than any other demographic with 54% of Asian-American teenagers reporting being bullied compared with 31.3% of white teens and 38.4% of black teens. In New York City, a report released in 2017 by the Asian American Legal Defense and Education Fund and The Sikh Coalition revealed that half of all Asian American students have been the target of bias-bullying and harassment - mirroring national statistics. Depressed with the situation for Asian American children, New York magazine's Wesley Yang says "that to be an Asian American means being not just good at math and playing the violin, but a mass of stifled, repressed, abused, conformist quasi-robots who simply do not matter socially or culturally."

On December 3, 2009 at South Philadelphia High School in the "City of Brotherly Love," a horrendous mass bullying attack occurred when 30 Asian students were attacked (13 sent to the hospital) by 70 black students. This tragic event led to President Barack Obama visiting the school to tell students "Life is precious and part of its beauty lies in its diversity. We shouldn't be embarrassed by the things that make us different. We should be proud of them." Accompanying President Obama was U.S. Secretary of Education Arne Duncan who said "From any difficult situation, you hope it never happens again. You have to deal with the issues openly and honestly and you have to be sure the district emerges stronger."

Before the massive attack, Asian students say black students routinely pelted them with food, punched, and kicked them in school hallways and bathrooms, and hurled racial slurs like "Hey, Chinese!" Vietnamese immigrant Duong Nghe Ly says "I thought America would be like the "Hannah Montana" TV episodes I had watched in Vietnam. What I found in Philadelphia was closer to "The Wire" so I kept my head down and tried to make my way through the broken system. I was often laughed at because of who I was. I went to school every day being scared, wondering when would be the next time I'd be attacked. My only goal is to study hard here so I can go to college and get a career to take care of my parents." During Ly's first week of school, he was robbed in the bathroom and his older brother was punched in the face. As to why black students acted violently, Ly says "Black students tell me they live in a violent environment with their parents having problems at home so they want to express their anger thru violence by attacking weak Asians."

Tyreke Williams, a black student at the school, upsettingly says "They're just hating on other races. They don't have anything better to do with their lives." Wali Smith, a black community specialist on anger management and conflict resolution, says "These black kids are scared cowards so will take advantage of weak Asian people. If blacks go to the bathroom and take Asian's money and Asians don't report it, they'll just keep riding it until the wheels fall off."

President of the Chinese American Student Association Wei Chen, who organized an eight-day boycott of the school with 50 students, said "We have suffered a lot to get to America. We just want a safe environment to learn. Getting assaulted hurt our bodies. It also hurt our hearts. I wish there is a place where racism doesn't exist." The boycott helped trigger national attention to the violence against Asian students at South Philly High School with a federal investigation launched following a formal civil rights complaint by the Asian American Legal Defense Fund and the Vietnamese embassy complaining to the U.S. Justice Department. Angered, Chief of the Justice Department's civil rights division Thomas Perez said "We intend to use every tool in our law enforcement arsenal to stamp out harassment and bullying in the schools. School districts are accountable for creating policies, practices and a climate of inclusion. If a school district deliberately ignores instances of harassment, they do so at their own peril. If we don't address bullying in middle school and high school, then we will foster a culture of intolerant adults."

Helen Gym, the first Asian-American Philadelphia City Council member, says "The focus of our federal complaint was never about problematic young people. It was truly the egregious conduct of school officials that warranted the federal intervention." A couple weeks later at a local NAACP meeting Helen said "It should have ended with DuBois, with King, with Malcolm, Rosa Parks, Cesar Chavez, with Yuri Kochiyama...To the School District: one issue which is not debatable is that the safety of our children is paramount and that violence against any one of our young people – no matter the color of our skin or what language we speak – can not and will not be tolerated. Dr. Martin Luther King, Jr. said: 'True peace is not the absence of tension but the presence of justice.' As we move forward, know that we are committed to the cause of justice not for any one group but for all the students of South Philadelphia High School."

After legal proceedings in 2010, Philadelphia's public school system accepted a consent decree aimed at curbing racial violence which subjects the school to state and federal oversight for 2.5 years. The school installed 126 security cameras, developed a plan for preventing bullying, conducted training to increase multicultural awareness, added more bilingual staffers, increased diversity training, and maintained records of harassment. A "50-50 club" took Asian and black students on group outings. The biggest addition was new principal Otis Hackney who said "As African-Americans, we can't forget our own struggle to the point that we become what we fought so hard against...There is no room for bullying at school. As principal, my No. 1 priority is to make sure my building is safe."

With bullying a huge concern across the country, Florida became the first state to offer bullied students vouchers up to $6,800 a year for private school tuition called the "Hope Scholarship Program" in 2018. Bullied students also have the option of moving to a different public school. In a statement Florida Governor Rick Scott said "Every child in Florida should have the opportunity to get a great education at the school of their choice so they can achieve their dreams." 50,000 students are bullied in Florida schools each year. The new voucher program, estimated to cost about $41 million, could provide as many as 5,800 students with vouchers.

ARMY HAZES ASIANS TO DEATH

With 1.4 million active U.S. military members, the United States has one of the largest armies in the world. There should be zero tolerance for bullying in the army.

Unfortunately in 2011, eight soldiers were charged in the suicide death of 19-year-old Chinese American infantryman Danny Chen who prosecutors say committed suicide by shooting himself after he was hazed, abused (assigned excessive guard duty to the point of exhaustion, knee kicked by soldiers while sitting), and subjected to ethnic slurs (Danny was called gook, chink, Jackie Chan, soy sauce, dragon lady, egg roll) for weeks at a remote combat outpost in southern Afghanistan. Specialist Nicholas Sepeda testified saying "Chen was unfairly singled out for punishment and ethnic harassment by his superiors, including Sgt. Adam Holcomb."

Hours before Danny committed suicide, he was forced to crawl on his belly across rocky gravel terrain for over 100 metres (330 feet) while fellow soldiers threw rocks at him. Danny wrote on his arms "Tell my parents I'm sorry" before committing suicide. In 2018, Danny Chen's mother Su Zhen Chen broke down emotionally when the tragic suicide event of her only child became an opera called "An American Soldier" by the composer Huang Ruo and the playwright David Henry Hwang.

Concerned that Chen's death is a reflection of a larger problem of military hazing, Sen. Kirsten Gillibrand, D-N.Y., a member of the Senate Armed Services Committee, called on the Defense Department to conduct a system-wide review of alleged hazing incidents in the military saying "I cannot imagine what Chen's parents are going through as they mourn the senseless loss of their son. No soldier should have to mentally or physically fear another soldier. There is no room for discrimination and mistreatment in our military. We need to ensure that those responsible for this type of abuse are held accountable and we must take steps to prevent any more tragedies from happening. It is outrageous that any man or woman serving our country would be subject to discrimination or harassment."

Earlier in the same year, 21-year-old U.S. Marine Corps Lance Corporal Harry Lew committed suicide (placed the muzzle of his M249 squad automatic weapon in his mouth and pulled the trigger) in his foxhole in Afghanistan after he was kicked and punched by fellow Marines. Before his death, Lew wrote on his arm "may hate me now, but in the long run this was the right choice, I'm sorry - my mom deserves the truth." According to an investigation, "Lew was subjected to a series of physical tasks, had sand dumped on his face, and was kicked and punched in the helmet, and forced to dig a fox hole to sleep in."

In 2012 at a congressional hearing on military hazing, Harry Lew's aunt Congresswoman Judy Chu said "It's a difficult matter to talk about in such a public setting. My nephew Lew was beaten and sand was poured on his face after he fell asleep while on guard. 22 minutes after they stopped abusing him, at 3:43 a.m., Harry climbed into a foxhole and killed himself with his own gun. And what punishment was given? Virtually nothing. In Harry's case, three Marines were charged, one Marine was given just one month in confinement, two were found not guilty by a jury of their peer fellow Marines." In response, Sgt. Maj. of the Marine Corps Michael Barrett told Congresswoman Chu "The small-unit leadership failed. I wish I could take it all back. We should have done better. But we are aggressively attacking these societal concerns as hard as we could possibly take them, and you have our assurance on that" and Sgt. Maj. of the Army Raymond Chandler III said "Let me give you the bottom line up front: Hazing has no place in our Army. We will not tolerate hazing in any form, and we will hold those in violation of this policy accountable for their actions." Chu was not impressed at the lip service.

4 years later in 2016, Rep Judy Chu introduced the "Harry Lew Military Hazing Accountability and Prevention Act" that requires the Department of Defense to create a national database of hazing incidents in the military and to submit an annual report on the DOD's actions to stop hazing through training and response. Bill co-sponsor Rep. Debbie Dingell (D-MI) says "We all have an obligation to bring more accountability to the system and improve training so hazing is tracked and handled appropriately. We owe it to those we've lost to take action to prevent more senseless tragedies from happening in the future."

Yet again, it is saddening to see society be reactive instead of proactive on preventing suicides thru bullying and racism.

POLICE ASIAN AMERICAN BRUTALITY

In 2012, Chicago Mayor Rahm Emanuel pledged to make Chicago "the most immigrant-friendly city in the world" with the "Welcoming City Ordinance" which prohibits city employees and police officers from asking law-abiding individuals about their immigration status or discriminate against them for their English speaking abilities. Following Chicago's lead, many cities across America such as Boston, Orlando, and Philadelphia have adopted similar laws. In 2016, the City of Chicago further strengthened the ordinance with an amendment that defined abuse to include verbal threats such as threatening deportation. The ordinance is extremely important as Asian Americans are often treated as "perpetual foreigners" even though Asian Americans are U.S. Citizens or on the path for citizenship due to non-Asians viewing Asians as a threat due to high education achievement rates and record as quality employees.

Unfortunately in 2013, Jianqing "Jessica" Klyzek, a Chinese-American woman U.S. citizen, was beaten by a group of Chicago police officers inside the Copper Tan and Spa for suspicion of running a prostitution ring. While telling the officers that she is a United States Citizen and does not engage in any illegal business practices, Officer Gerald DiPasquale verbally abused Jessica by saying "You're not f—— American! I'll put you in a UPS box and send you back to wherever the f— you came from! No, you're not a citizen! You're here on our borrowed time. So mind your f—— business before I shut this whole f—— place down. And I'll take this place and then whoever owns it will f—— kill you because they don't care about you, OK? I'll take this building. You'll be dead and your family will be dead." Another officer struck Jessica in the head as she was handcuffed on the ground. After seeing footage of the disturbing police brutality on a law-abiding Asian American women citizen, Asian American activists stormed to Chicago Mayor Rahm Emanuel's office at the City Hall. Attorney Nebula Li, who handles police brutality cases, says "Some may find it shocking to hear those words coming out of a Chicago police officer's mouth, but many of us in the Asian-American community have been told all our lives that we don't belong and to go back to wherever we came from." Activists also posted flyers throughout Chinatown featuring Jessica's battered face to raise awareness about police brutality against Asian Americans. The Spa owner sued the Chicago police department of committing hate crime for stereotyping that Asian Americans are second-class citizens and don't belong in America, excessive use of physical force instead of handling issues judiciously thru law, and falsifying the circumstances of her arrest (prostitution ring). The Asian Americans Advancing Justice (AAAJ) group called the suspensions inadequate saying "The entire incident was caught on video. The things that the officers were saying to Jessica were really upsetting and hit a historical nerve in the Asian-American community."

ASIAN BUSINESS TARGETING

As the FBI reports, Asian business owners are often labelled as "easy targets" because they are perceived to speak limited English and won't reach out to law enforcement for help.

In 2014, 49-year-old prominent lawyer Danford Grant, a married man with three children, was sentenced to 25 years in prison for raping five Asian women at a series of Asian massage parlors in the Seattle area. Grant was described by police as a serial rapist who was obsessed with Asian women - particularly immigrant Asian American masseuses who couldn't speak English and would feel shameful about reporting rape. He chose his Asian American massage therapist rape targets by researching their personal information beforehand and booking appointments under false names with burner phones. Grant was caught fleeing from his fifth rape when police found a pistol, bag of Viagra, a computer with internet search histories of "rape scenes," and his wedding ring in his Honda Pilot car. What's scary is that Grant acted polite saying he was an attorney, police officer, or doctor and then lied about his wife being dead before raping the women who refused to have sex with him. Shocked, the fifth rape victim said "I'm particularly fearful of the ones who appear well-mannered and friendly because they would remind me of the bastard who tried to rape me. I cannot use a small knife in the kitchen because it looks similar to the knife Grant used to rape me."

In 2017, the FBI arrested individuals responsible for a recent series of at least 9 violent commercial robberies targeting Asian owned businesses, restaurants, and salons in Atlanta Georgia. Per the FBI, "The robberies all appear to have been committed by males approximately 5'08" – 6'00", with thin builds, in their late teens to mid-twenties. Two suspects generally enter the businesses, often initially acting as customers, while a third serves as a getaway driver."

In 2019, 51-year old Vietnamese Ngoc Nguyen, mother of three and grandmother of two, was killed by 21-year-old Krystal Whipple, who drove over Ngoc's body by car, when she ran away from paying a $35 manicure bill at a Las Vegas Nail Salon.

ASIAN FAMILIES ROBBED BY GUNPOINT

Many Asian Americans experience racism in public by racists who are conditioning to view Asians as inferior perpetual foreigners by their parents, friends, media portrayal, celebrities, and all other forms of media that portray damaging Asian stereotypes.

Since 2016, the Sacramento Police Department said they sent out an alert via NextDoor warning South Sacramento residents of increases in armed robberies targeting Asians of which 400 homes have been victims. Police said several robberies happened while the victims were at home getting out of their car where the suspects were following them by car days before. The thieves' assumption is that Asian victims don't speak English so won't fight back and won't report to the police. Peter Chung described his horrifying experience saying "Two armed men kicked down the front door of my home and held me, my brother and my mother hostage at gunpoint. The men then forced us into a car to withdraw $8,000 from a bank." 46-year-old Hua Cai Chen, who was shot in the calf and robbed of $700 in cash by two men as he exited his car, sadly says "Sacramento is too scary. I don't know how to live now. I have a mortgage to pay, a wife and child to feed." Sacramento residents such as Kent Tran says "I'm shocked. I've actually armed myself with weapons and stun guns, a surveillance system, and upped my security system with glass-break sensors." Tom Phung, who has lived in Sacramento for over 35 years, says "We have nearly a dozen families who have moved out of Sacramento, even selling their house below cost just to get the hell out. In this neighborhood, there's a gun pointed or fired almost every night. The police takes 40-50 minutes to arrive." The community has organized a WeChat group of 500 members to report suspicious activities where members who speak English can translate the crime to police.

There have also been robberies targeting Asian communities in Philadelphia Pennsylvania where Ivan Zhou, whose father was robbed at gunpoint by three men, says "Our community has a lot of immigrants, individuals who don't speak native English. Everyday there's a new case. Everyone is just crossing their fingers, hoping that it will just all end." In 2017 for the crimes in Philadelphia, U.S. District Judge Petrese Tucker sentenced Tyree Mansell to 36 years and eight months in federal prison for a string of 2015 home-invasion robberies against Asians with the Judge saying "This defendant is a violent recidivist. The defendant has no respect for the law."

Raleigh Asian business owners were also terrorized at their homes in 2018 when 22-year old Jun Wang, who owns three Chinese restaurants in the area, was robbed by three masked and gloved Spanish speaking men. Jun says his biggest lesson is "Close and lock the door first before turning off the home alarm system so that no one can sneak in undetected. Keep your cash in the bank and carry just plastic credit cards that can be cancelled." In the same year owner of China Wok Hong Zheng was killed outside his home during a robbery in nearby Durham North Carolina. This saddened many in the North Carolina triangle community who knew Hong as a friend. In self-defense to protect their families, about 100 Asian business owners have banned together to form the North Carolina Chinese Hunting Club to train in shooting techniques once a month at the Wake County Firearms Education & Training Center with instructor Wei Miao.

Raleigh restaurant owner Lang Dong says "I don't leave my home without strapping a 9mm semi-automatic Glock 17 pistol to my hip. My wife and I own seven guns: three pistols, one AR-15 and one shotgun in the restaurant as well as another pair at home. My wife keeps a pistol in her purse. If there's a car directly behind me on my way home, I'll keep going because don't want to risk leading them to my family. I've also installed a steel-plated panic room in my house and instruct my children to bolt themselves behind the reinforced door in case of an attack."

In addition to life-threatening armed robberies, Asian Americans are racially abused. In 2018 in Fremont California, a U.S. Air Force Reserve James Ahn was racially abused by a woman who stated that James wasn't driving fast enough when he was driving at the legal speed limit. In the viral Facebook video, the woman said to James "This is not your f-ing country, this is my country. Go back to f--ing China, you ugly Chinese" while making a derogatory slanted eyes gesture. Angered U.S. Representative Eric Swalwell tweeted "I proudly represent #Fremont in Congress. This woman does not represent Fremont, which is a diverse, inclusive community. But she's a reminder of the hate that still exists in America and the work we all have ahead. Thank you, James Ahn, for your service to America."

In 2017, 21-year-old Vietnamese college male Henry Nguyen was enjoying time with his girlfriend at the OC Night Market until a white couple punched Henry in the face while yelling "Go back to Asia. Go eat Dog!" for Henry refusing to let the white couple cut a long line everyone else was patiently waiting in. When Henry and his girlfriend left the market at 11PM, the White couple had been stalking them all day so pulled up next to Henry's car to break his teeth and bloody his face before speeding away. Stunned, Henry said "I was just thinking, all this could've been avoided if they just got in line. She didn't have to be racist." Saddened to see the racism, OC Night Market organizer said "Our event is a platform that celebrates diversity and all cultures in our community and every event draws a more diverse crowd. We are happy the victims are on their way to recovery and hope that law enforcement will be able to sort this out." His girlfriend raised $6,413 on GoFundMe to pay for his emergency room visit and dental work on his teeth.

CHAPTER 4

OVERCOMING ASIAN DISCRIMINATION

No one is born hating another person because of the color of his skin or his background or his religion."

- President Barack Obama quoting Nelson Mandela (most liked tweet in Twitter's history in response to 2012 Charlottesville Violence)

RACISM AND DISCRIMINATION

I've faced racism and discrimination my entire life - bullied for being Asian, dumb, short, unathletic, poor, shy, skinny, and fat. Counted out my whole life, I thrive on the underdog role to succeed in honor of my family name "Huynh" pronounced "win."

Growing up in the State of Maine, my brother, myself, mom, and dad were the earliest Asians to settle in Maine as my parents were sponsored by a Catholic Priest from Waterville, Maine to pursue the American Dream as boat people from the Vietnam War. Since the early 1980s to this day, my mom still works at a press laundry and father still works at a semiconductor company making silicon wafers - all blue collar jobs. Despite low income jobs, my parents promised each other to be fiscally responsible in saving the majority of their income so that my younger brother and I could achieve the "American Dream" thru getting good grades and accomplishments in grade school that would lead to obtaining degrees from the best colleges in the world for great careers with comfortable salaries needed to raise a family.

As a first generation Asian American born in South Portland, Maine from parents who risked their lives as "boat people" escaping Vietnam re-education camp as South Vietnamese Army Prisoners of War, I faced and still face countless discrimination in America. Many tap into faith to overcome challenges. I tapped into fitness.

I've faced and embraced the challenges of being a trailblazer in our family such as being the first to graduate college, first to get a white collar job, first to live in the ghetto twice, first to sleep on an airbed for 6 consecutive years (consulting and business school), first to complete Master's degree, and first to turn down six figure careers in pursuing my fitness passion via entrepreneurship.

Despite these achievements, most people don't know that I spoke broken English until Age 10 - getting pulled out of class 3 hours everyday to attend the school's "English as a Second Language (ESL)" program. Outside of class, I tried to learn English by watching "Dragon Ball Z." As the only Asian in school and basically the entire state of Maine as Maine is the whitest state in the United States where 95% of the population is white and 1% is Asian, I was always made fun of for my accent, squinty eyes, nerdiness, weak physical abilities, and skin color.

ASIAN RACISM THRU LIFE

Hollywood and the media have the biggest influences on how Asian Americans are treated in the United States as family's perceptions are shaped by what they "see" at the movie theatres or on television and "hear" from the media or public gossip. From before I was born in 1988 to now in 2018, Asian men have been emasculated as weak, nerdy outcasts, and shy losers who can't attract women whereas women are portrayed as people who speak broken English and are submissive to men.

With the capture of South Vietnam by the Communist North Vietnamese in 1975 after the United States pulled all soldiers out of the war, Hollywood capitalized on the war - producing numerous blockbuster $100 million films including "Platoon" in 1986 starring Charlie Sheen, "Full Metal Jacket" in 1987 starring Ronald Ermey as Sergeant Hartman, and "Good Morning, Vietnam" in 1987 starring Robin Williams as a radio DJ on Armed Forces Radio Service.

In"Full Metal Jacket," there are two scenes that degrade Vietnamese women with the lines "me so horny...me love you long time...me sucky sucky" when a prostitute approached two American soldier for sex and "you boys want #1 f--ky? she give you everything you want, long time" when a pimp was negotiating the prostitute price with an army platoon. From these two scenes, many white men develop an "Asian fetish" towards Asian women with the hope of a submissive wife who will not talk back, cooks, and can fulfill their sexual desires at night.

American men continue to have the perception that Asian women are "easy to get" due to Asian nations historically pleasing American soldiers during wartime to prevent American soldiers from raping women living in occupied territories at the end of World War II. In China after World War II,

President Chiang Kai-shek encouraged 54,000 U.S. marines to stay by opening 450 cafes, dance clubs, and restaurants near the military bases where Marine Lt. Carl Johnson wrote a letter to his wife describing Tianjin as "The village itself consists of about thirty bars and cafes. Each one is a house of prostitution and there is nothing undercover about it." After the United States occupied Japan in 1945, Japanese officials created the "Recreation and Amusement Association (RAA)" to provide "comfort facilities" in preventing rape by American troops because an estimated 10,000 women were raped by Allied military troops in Okinawa Japan during World War II. RAA Chief of Public Relation Seiichi Kaburagi said "Over 4 months, there were 70,000 Japanese prostitutes serving 350,000 U.S. troops in Japan. 1 Japanese women had sex with 47 American troops each day for $2 USD total." U.S. General Douglas MacArthur shut down the brothels in 1946 amid complaints from military chaplains about the "R&R Rest & Recreation or I&I Intoxication & Intercourse" offerings. In South Korea during the 1960s, South Korean President Park Chung-hee created "prostitution towns" where over 350,000 women served U.S. troops that accounted for 25% of South Korea's GNP.

Personally, my grade school classmates would make fun of my small eyes by "pulling their eyes back" and say "you sucky sucky" - bullying me for my broken English, shy personality, and weak physique. Students would ask what my mom was making for dinner saying "hey Ching Chong, your momma making chicken fried rice tonight?!" During recess I was never picked to play soccer with bullies saying "American doesn't want you here, go back to Vietnam and work in a Nike sweatshop."

In "Good Morning, Vietnam," U.S. Army radio host Robin Williams on one of his segments said "What is a demilitarized zone? It sounds like something out of the Wizard of Oz...Oh look you've landed in Saigon, you're among the little people now." This is yet another example of discrimination against Asian men for being short which leads to women not even wanting to consider dating Asian men, sports scouts not paying attention to Asian athletes, Hollywood not casting Asians in lead roles, and corporate America excluding Asians from leadership opportunities because Asians don't fit the "tall white men" demographic.

From 1998-2007, which was when I was ages 10-19 going thru middle school and high school, Jackie Chan collaborated with Chris Tucker in the "Rush Hour" trilogy. Jackie Chan tried to carry on Bruce Lee's action movie legacy by collaborating with non-Asian actors such as Bruce Lee did with white martial artist Chuck Norris in "Way of the Dragon" in 1972, black martial artist Jim Kelly in "Enter the Dragon" in 1973, and black basketball star Kareem Abdul-Jabbar in "Game of Death" in 1978. Similarly in America, Jackie Chan helped propel the career of black actor Chris Tucker in the "Rush Hour" trilogy where Chris Tucker made $25 million + 20% of box office sales ($258 million box office) in "Rush Hour 3." And Jackie Chan also launched the career of white actor Owen Wilson in the first of three movies together called "Shanghai Noon" in 2000 that helped Owen star in movies "Zoolander," "Behind Enemy Lines, "Wedding Crashers," and "Cars 3."

In "Rush Hour 1" when Chris Tucker meets Jackie Chan for the first time at the airport he says "Please tell me you speak English, I'm Detective Carter...Do you understand the words that are coming out of my mouth! I cannot believe this s**t! First I get a bulls**t assignment. Now Mr. Rice-a-roni. Don't even speak American." This scene captures how Asian Americans who speak broken English or don't want to engage with racist people get treated in America.

In "Rush Hour 2" when speaking with black actor Don Cheadle, Chris Tucker says "You're embarrassing yourself, you're a black man with a Chinese restaurant...alright uc-taw it-ah oop-ta oom-ski." When I travelled to New Orleans with my wife, many black men kept asking if I was "blackinese" in exact reference to this scene.

In "Rush Hour 3" when Chris Tucker catches up with Jackie Chan, Chris says "That's right Lee. For the last 3 years I have studied the ancient teaching of Buddha - earning 2 black belts in Wushu martial arts...I am half Chinese baby." Nelson Mandela said we should treat all people with respect instead of engaging in cultural appropriation.

Two years after "Rush Hour 3" came "The Hangover" trilogy from 2009-2013, while I was ages 21-24, featuring Asian American Ken Jeong as Leslie Chow. Ken was portrayed speaking with a broken English accent, weak, small penis, short, and small eyes. Hollywood did not portray Leslie Chow in a positive hero-like role that can inspire men to be strong and sexy.

In 2014, 1 year later and 2 years after the Facebook IPO, Hollywood produced a TV show called "Silicon Valley" with an Asian character named Jian-Yang played by Jimmy O. Yang. Jian-Yang is portrayed as someone who speaks broken English, is nerdy, and can never attract women due to his awkwardness and weak physique. People who follow the show especially women tend to assume that Asian men are not physically and socially attractive.

PERPETUAL FOREIGNER ASIAN STEREOTYPE

In America, Asian Americans are generally not considered Americans even though they have U.S. Citizenship or Green Card holders but are instead viewed as "perpetual foreigners." As mentioned, stereotypes of Asian Americans are often portrayed in the media, literature, internet, film, television, and music which shape society's perception for hate crimes.

During the 1870s after the Civil War, California political leaders blamed Chinese laborers for the low wages saying "the Chinese are a perpetual, unchanging, and unchangeable alien element that can never become homogeneous; that their civilization is demoralizing and degrading to our people; that they degrade and dishonor labor; and they can never become citizens" which led to President Chester Arthur signing into federal law the Chinese Exclusion Act in 1882 that prohibited immigration of Chinese laborers. Historically, the Chinese Exclusion Act was the first law ever to prevent people from an ethnic group from immigrating into the U.S. Chinese immigrants were prohibited from owning property and barred from working in most industries aside from hand-laundry and restaurant businesses resulting in Chinese immigrants forced to make a living thru self-employment with men working in restaurants and women in garment factories.

Anti-slavery politicians were upset such as Massachusetts senator George Frisbie Hoar who said "The Chinese Exclusion Act is nothing less than the legalization of racial discrimination meant to retain white superiority especially with regards to working privileges." Racism towards Chinese was at an all-time high in Rock Springs Wyoming in 1885 when 150 armed white miners kicked Chinese immigrants out of town by burning their homes and businesses while murdering 28 people - none of the white miners were charged in the murders. Fearful for their lives, Chinese immigrants moved east (Boston, Philadelphia, New York) to escape violence by seeking safety in numbers in neighborhoods known today as "Chinatowns." Per Indiana University History Professor Ellen Wu, "Beginning in the late 19th century and really through the 1940s and 1950s, there was what we can call a regime of Asian exclusion: a web of laws and social practices designed to shut out Asians completely from American life. That's really how Chinatowns came into being as a way to contain a very threatening population in American life." The Chinese Exclusion Act was abolished in 1952.

From 1942-1946 during World War II, 120,000 Japanese Americans living in Western United States were forced into concentration camps by President Franklin D. Roosevelt. The Commission on Wartime Relocation and Internment of Civilians (CWRIC) report, titled "Personal Justice Denied," found zero evidence of Japanese American disloyalty during World War II and concluded that the incarceration had been the product of racism - recommending the government pay reparations to the 120,000 internees. In 1988, President Ronald Reagan signed into law the Civil Liberties Act of 1988 which apologized for the internment on behalf of the U.S. government and approved a $20,000 payment to each internee survivor ($1.6 billion in total) with the U.S. Government admitting their actions were based on "race prejudice, war hysteria, and a failure of political leadership."

My mom is 100% Chinese DNA whose parents moved from China to Chinese section of South Vietnam called Cho Lon and my dad is 25% Chinese / 75% Vietnamese with his father 50% Chinese making me 62.5% Chinese and 37.5% Vietnamese. Cultured in both ethnicities and more fluent speaking in Vietnamese, I'm still treated as a "perpetual foreigner" where people tell me to "go back to China" in public, at school, and work.

BEAT UNATHLETIC COMMENTS WITH GOATS

Many Asians aren't born with athletic genetics, which is why you don't see many Asians making a living like LeBron James shooting basketballs thru a hole or The Rock starring in blockbuster movies, so it's hard to develop an athletic physique without the right knowledge and motivation - knowing your physique is 30% genetic and 70% from lifestyle. As a child, I was discriminated against for being unathletic due to being skinny then fat, short, shy, and weak.

Being fat and weak was very tough mentally and emasculating while I was in grade school, college, and work. Getting fat shamed, losing out on business deals, not being able to attract desirable love mates, and being viewed as an outcast from social circles are all low points that I experienced while fat and weak. The only way to enjoy the benefits of being physically strong and athletic is by exercising and focusing on proper nutrition.

As a child with a max height of 5 foot 2 inches, I was always the shortest person - never picked for pickup sports games in basketball, soccer, or flag football due to my unathleticism and being fat. I wasn't able to make friends as I stood alone sadly watching classmates have fun while no one would play with me. Seeing the mental toll I experienced from being physically weak, my father enrolled my brother and I in martial arts at Age 12 while also joining the middle school track team. The combination of martial arts and power athletics is the foundation of JustHuynh fitness today.

For motivation to stay committed and overcome two more bouts with obesity during college and work, I look up to three athletic icons who succeeded by "playing angry with a chip on their shoulder to become the GOAT (greatest of all time) in their sport."

Growing up watching dubbed over Chinese movies, I was exposed to Eurasian martial artist Bruce Lee who was a role model for Asian men who have been emasculated as skinny, weak, and shy. Bruce was driven to succeed when Hollywood directors told him he couldn't star in an American film because "American audiences are only comfortable with white actors and actresses. Starring an actor of Asian descent would not result in good box office sales." Bruce Lee made Asian men "sexy" again with his famous shirtless fighting scenes - being called the greatest martial artists ever and "the Father of Mixed Martial Arts." Many children started enrolling in martial arts.

Not knowledgeable about how to play sports due to my family not in the know about youth sports, I was fortunate to have run across my second favorite athlete who "plays angry with a chip on their shoulder" named Michael Jordan who starred in the "Space Jam" basketball movie. Michael Jordan always reminds himself about being cut from the high school varsity basketball team because he was "too short" at 5 feet 11 inches. This motivated Michael to prove the doubters wrong by winning 6 NBA Championships during the 1990s - being viewed as the greatest basketball player of all-time where children wanted to "be like Mike" and wear #23.

Motivated by Bruce Lee and Michael Jordan about the benefits of being fit, I committed to martial arts and track for the next 8 years which helped me improve physically as one of the best martial artists at my dojo and sprinters on the track team as captain. I also improved intellectually to gain admission into an elite college in Bowdoin College and was no longer bullied.

Then in college, I experienced the "College Freshman 15" where I got fat by drinking alcohol and eating unhealthy food. Being fat impacted me negatively where I was not viewed as attractive by women, performed poorer academically, and got weaker athletically.

In need of motivation, I encountered my third favorite athlete who "plays angry with a chip on their shoulder" named Tom Brady of the New England Patriots. Tom Brady's drive to succeed is from being drafted #199 in the 2000 NFL Draft and starting out as the 4th string quarterback. He puts a reminder of being picked #199 in his locker room. From 2001 to 2019, Tom Brady has won 5 NFL Championships that has changed his life professionally being recognized as the greatest football player of all-time and personally in gaining the love of Brazilian supermodel Gisele Bundchen. What makes Brady successful is his attention to detail studying an opponent on film and turning practice repetitions into game reality where he feels comfortable leading his team to victory from a 4th quarter deficit. Time and time again, Brady and Coach Belichick eliminate the opponent's strength and attack their weaknesses. Brady's top five games are in Super Bowl 36 when he defeated the Rams' "Greatest Show on Turf" offense, 2007's 16-0 Perfect Season, Super Bowl 49 defeating Seattle's "Legion of Boom" defense, Super Bowl 51 coming back from 28-3 against the Atlanta Falcons' Matt Ryan trying to take Brady's "Quarterback Throne," and 2019 AFC Championship Game victory on the road against Kansas City's #1 Offense in front of 70,000 fans rooting against the Patriots while Patrick Mahomes wanted to be "King of the NFL." Just as people wanted to look great like Bruce Lee shirtless or like Michael Jordan dunking basketballs, people wanted to wear the #12 jersey and win championships like Tom Brady.

Motivated as an underdog, I recommitted to martial arts and sprinting that helped me get healthier, improve my economics grade, and land a management consulting job with PwC.

As a consultant after graduation, I went thru my third time being fat as I didn't exercise and ate terribly due to living in hotels 200 nights a year over 4 years. I suffered personally being unattractive to potential loves, athletically by having an obese BMI, and professionally not being respected in business meetings due to my weight. I recall one moment where I tried tight business clothes on and had the most embarrassing moment in life when the buttons of my dress shirt and back of my pants wanted to rip from sitting.

I didn't want to suffer being a loser and loner past my thirties so committed to martial arts and fitness again after seeing Tom Brady still motivated in his 30s even with Super Bowl championships and a supermodel wife. This inspired me to improve professionally obtaining my Vanderbilt MBA and launching JustHuynh Fitness to help people boost confidence, be healthy, and improve self defense thru martial arts and power athletics. Athletically, people continue to underestimate me for being short and Asian where I'm able to prove them wrong by being faster on the track, better on the sportsfield, and lethal in martial arts. On a personal front, women want to marry men who can "provide and protect" like Kevin Hart said in his "I'm Not a Fighter" comedy skit. My wife loves me for my ability to "protect" her as a skilled martial artist and "provide" as an entrepreneur.

TEASED FOR BEING DUMB

Throughout my life, I've been teased for being an idiot, my broken English, and assumption that I have low business acumen due to being a child of blue collar Asian parents.

From grade school to middle school, I was teased for being pulled out of normal class everyday for 2 hours in the "English as a Second Language (ESL)" program. Some classmates whispered "have fun in ESL camp Asia boy" in reference to the Chinese being forced into Chinatowns and Japanese being placed in internment camps during World War II.

Entering high school, I was disrespected by my 8th grade guidance counselor - being placed in the "special education" 9th grade English class reserved for the lowest performing 20 out of 220 students. Motivated to prove people wrong in achieving the American Dream thru education, I graduated with the 8th highest academic ranking out of 220 students - being admitted into Bowdoin College.

As a management consultant, I faced the "bamboo ceiling" where I was passed over for promotions and high-profile assignments. I had to overcome preconceptions thru my execution where people apologized for thinking I was not capable of performing at a high level.

It is also good to keep in mind that you don't have to be a graduate of Harvard University, MIT, or Stanford University to be successful. In business, shiny degrees don't matter as its all about providing the best solution for your customers. Three entrepreneurs who I admire are Sam Walton of Walmart (University of Missouri) who built a global retail chain from a suburban upbringing, Steve Jobs of Apple (Reed College) who changed the world with the phone and computers, and Harland Sanders of KFC (La Salle Extension University) who persevered in selling his fried chicken recipe despite being rejected 1,009 consecutive times.

DISRESPECTED FOR BEING YOUNG

In business, office politics get in the way when managers and leaders put down talented young professionals in favor of older and unqualified professionals. This is a huge reason why many organizations don't reach their full potential when office politics gets in the way of merit. Like sports, the best organizations have a "rank and yank" philosophy in making performance-based talent decisions.

Being young and feeling young is advantageous. You're always hungry, fresh, and motivated to succeed. Jeff Bezos, the world's only living $100 billion man as of November 2017, asks his team to embrace an "It's Always Day 1 at Amazon" approach to stay hungry in providing the best value for customers.

If you're being discriminated for being young, use these young stars in politics, business, and athletics. In politics, Theodore Roosevelt was the youngest U.S. President at 41 years 10 months old. In business, Mark Zuckerberg of Facebook became the youngest billionaire ever at age 23 in 2008. In sports, Tom Brady the #199 pick became the youngest quarterback to win the Super Bowl at age 24 - being known as the best NFL draft pick of all time.

BATTLING SUICIDAL THOUGHTS

Being discriminated against for being Asian, unattractive, weak, short, unsuccessful, dumb, shy, poor, and fat has led to dangerous suicidal thoughts.

In grade school, I overcame suicidal thoughts from racism with martial arts and track that helped me become disciplined, respectful, intelligent, driven, and athletic. My focus on achieving the American Dream thru obtaining top grades helped me ignore the haters.

In college, I overcame depression from not fitting in with the "cool kids" due to being short and Asian by knowing that there is world of opportunity outside of the college "campus bubble." I got this perspective when studied abroad in megacity Sydney, Australia.

During my first four years of professional life as a management consultant with PwC, I was depressed for being passed over for promotion twice given my contributions leading a team of 1,000 people on the historic $1 billion Independent Foreclosure Review project where banks had to revamp their policies following the 2008 Mortgage Crisis. Meeting my wife in 2012 gave me perspective that travelling for work was not sustainable and I needed to find a passion worth waking up for in the morning. As such, I left consulting to pursue my MBA degree at Vanderbilt University.

During second year of business school, I was depressed when Sprint didn't make a full-time offer after my summer internship especially after proposing to my wife in Kansas City thinking we would start a family in Kansas City after graduation. This made second year of MBA tough as the majority of tech companies made offers to summer interns. When interviewing, I felt discriminated against as recruiters only phone-screened me to meet their quotas for "Asians interviewed." Although I didn't get my dream company Samsung's full-time job offer, I was thankful for a summer internship opportunity with Samsung's Director of Customer Service Ted Lee - that was ironically offered on April Fools Day in 2016 while I was waiting for a full-time $120,000 offer from Microsoft. To avoid the death scenario of turning down Samsung's internship offer and being surprisingly rejected by Microsoft's full-time offer, I pulled my candidacy from Microsoft and accepted Samsung's summer internship. This ended a nerve-racking second year as I was the last in my MBA class to get a job offer despite being one of the most qualified professionals and top scholars.

During my 12 week Samsung internship in the summer of 2016 after completing my MBA, I married my wife and envisioned raising a family in New Jersey with a $120,000 salary. After delivering one of the best summer internship presentations to Samsung executives, I was not immediately made an offer so drove back to Boston. This was depressing as my MBA classmates were making $150,000 at Amazon and my plans to start a family was halted.

The best entrepreneurs start companies thru personal pains and mine was the hazards fat does to you. While working out at the YMCA, my entrepreneurial light bulb lit up when I noticed people dreading their workouts. I realized my calling in life is help people thrive in life thru martial arts and power athletics. In December 2016, Samsung and the FBI both made six figure offers when I was committed to JustHuynh Fitness. Even though I wasn't making any revenue, I made the difficult decision with the support of my wife and family that making financial sacrifices now would be worth it where we can wake up happy changing people's lives thru fitness.

Without the unexpected break, I would never have transitioned from employee to entrepreneur. I highly encourage everyone take a long vacation to think about your purpose in life especially if you can offer a product or service that solves customer's pains.

As an entrepreneur, many have aspirations of immediate success like Mark Zuckerberg who became the youngest billionaire ever at age 23 doing what he loves, marrying his college friend, raising a family, and starting a charity, but entrepreneurship is not that easy. Paired with seeing less educated people like music stars, athletes, and movie stars make millions doing what they love at such a young age, I occasionally get depressed with nothing to show for my hard work and elite education from Bowdoin and Vanderbilt.

Since 4:44AM is my wakeup time for the gym, there have been times where I thought about committing suicide by veering off the highway at 70 miles per hour to fall 100 feet down to the highway below. Blessed, I feel there is an angel in my head during the darkest seconds of my life telling me that I must live for my wife and family and that there are over 2 billion overweight people in the world that I am destined to help thru JustHuynh Fitness' martial arts and power athletics. If you're suffering from depression with suicidal thoughts, I hope you have a supportive husband or wife, parents, and potential customers who motivate you to continue living.

CHAPTER 5

Asian Martial Arts Influences

A journey of a thousand miles begins with a single step

- Laozi

BUDDHISM: FAITH & FITNESS

Exercise helps connect your spiritual and physical wellness. Similar to going to church, temple, mosques, synagogues, or your place of worship, being fit helps you carry out your life purpose. Buddha taught the importance of a strong body, saying "To keep the body in good health is a duty… otherwise we shall not be able to keep our mind strong and clear."

To conquer your fear of exercise, Buddhist Thich Nhat Hanh reminds us that "People have a hard time letting go of their suffering...you must have courage...courage is not the absence of fear, it is the mastery of it." Remember fear is just a state of mind. You'll dominate once can courageous achieve what you set your mind to. Buddha says you can break your own limitations as "The mind is everything. What you think, you become."

Fitness is a journey as there is no overnight quick fix. Buddha reminds us that "A jug fills drop by drop" meaning you must stay committed.

MARTIAL ARTS

If you follow Bruce Lee or Jackie Chan, you know Asians are famous for being martial artists. Asians love martial arts for the anti-ageing benefits, self defense skills, lower obesity risks, and improved mental health. From Chinese Kung Fu to Japanese Karate to Korean Taekwondo to Thai Kickboxing, and many additional martial arts styles, all help you thrive personally, physically, and professionally. As you develop your own self defense style, it's important to be familiar with Asia's impact on martial arts around the world. You'll notice that most martial arts were formed due to self defense needs against bullies or enemies.

FIVE ELDERS OF SHAOLIN - 581 AD

Shaolin Buddhist Monks are the guardians of Kung Fu martial arts who train in kung fu for self-defense against bullies and bandits. In Hollywood, the most famous Kung Fu practitioners are Bruce Lee, his master IP Man, Gordon Liu, Jackie Chan, Sammo Hung, Jet Li, Donnie Yen, Michael Jai White, Wu Jing (Wolf Warrior), Ray Park, Scott Adkins, Robert Downey Jr. ("Ironman" movies), Christian Bale (Batman) and Michelle Waterson (UFC Fighter). In 1993, Jason Scott Lee famously portrayed Bruce Lee in the martial arts film "Dragon: The Bruce Lee Story" and in 2012 documented his training at Shaolin in the documentary "Secrets of Shaolin with Jason Scott Lee." Some of the best Kung Fu movies are "Five Shaolin Masters" featuring David Chiang; "Enter the Dragon," "Fist of Fury," and "The Chinese Connection" featuring Bruce Lee; "The 36th Chamber of Shaolin," "Clan of the White Lotus," and "Right Diagram Pole Fighter" featuring Gordon Liu; "Snake in the Eagle's Shadow" and "Drunken Master" featuring Jackie Chan; "The Invincible Armour" featuring Hwang Jang Lee, "The Shaolin Temple" featuring Jet Li, "Five Deadly Venoms" featuring Chiang Sheng; "The Prodigal Son," and "Warriors Two" starring Sammo Hung; "Ip Man" featuring Donnie Yen, and "Fatal Contact" featuring Wu Jing.

For over 1,000 years, Shaolin kept their distance from the Chinese government until the Qing Dynasty defeated the Ming Dynasty in China. In defense of the Ming in 1673, 128 Shaolin monks defeated Qing's army of without suffering a single casualty. Worried of the Shaolin monks resistance in 1723, Qing sent an army outnumbering the monks 10:1 that killed 110 of the 128 monks. 70 days later, only 5 of the surviving 18 monks remained - Ng Mui, Jee Sin Sim See, Bak Mei, Fung Dou Dak, and Miu Hin. The Five Elders martial arts have been passed down to current martial artists. This massacre is on par with "Star Wars" Anakin Skywalker turning to the "dark side of the force" in murdering skilled Jedi in the Jedi Temple.

Ng Mui's most famous lineage of martial artists are IP man and his student Bruce Lee. Ng Mui started teaching Wing Chun, Dragon Style, and White Crane when she saved a 15-year-old girl from a bandit who was trying to force her into marriage. Ng Mui made Wing Chun easy to learn without the need for physical strength - making Ng Mui's style female-friendly.

Reverend Master Leader Jee Sin Sim See is famous for training folk hero Wong Fei Hung and his father. When the leader of the Shaolin Temple Hong Mei ("Red Eyebrows") died, Jee Sin Sim See became leader and Bak Mei was upset because Jee Sin Sim See's loyalty was to the Ming dynasty. As such, Bak Mei left the monks to join the Qing Army and returned once more to Shaolin to kill Jee Sin Sim See by breaking his neck.

Bak Mei is the most famous of the Fiver Elders known as the "Taoist with White Eyebrows" played by Gordon Liu in the "Kill Bill" film. As a traitor and now member of the Qing Army, Bak Mei trained 50,000 Imperial troops. For revenge, Bak Mei died of poisoning by martial artists.

Fung Dou Dak saved herbal medicine manuals and escaped through a secret tunnel during the Shaolin massacre. To avoid being caught as a Buddhist by the Qing Army, Fung Dou Dak converted to Taoism.

Miu Hin is the father of Miu Tsui Fa and the grandfather of folk hero Fong Sai-Yuk. After escaping the Qing Army massacre, Bak Mei wanted more political involvement and more students while the other four elders favored the opposite. The disagreement led to a duel between Jee Sin and Bak Mei - resulting in the death of Jee Sin. Angered by Jee Sin's death, Miu Hin challenged Bak Mei but was also killed. After observing Bak Mei's techniques in killing Jee Sin and Miu Hin, Fung Dou Dak challenged Bak Mei to a final duel - defeating Bak Mei who later died from injuries and poisoning.

KARATE - GICHIN FUNAKOSHI 1372

Karate began in the 14th century in Okinawa and became mainstream in the 1920s when Gichin Funakoshi introduced karate into mainland Japan beginning in Tokyo. Unarmed combat techniques developed when King Shō Shin banned weapons in 1477. Karate's techniques come from Chinese Kung Fu - particularly Fujian White Crane.

As a teenager, Gichin Funakoshi (born in 1868) was sick and weak. Fortunately Gichin was in the same class as the son of karate master Yasutsune Azato. Funakoshi was Azato's only student who taught at night as the government forbid the teaching of karate - viewing the hands and feet as "weapons" against government authority. Gichin also learned martial arts from Yasutsune Itosu and Itosu's master Sokon Matsumura.

In 1922, Gichin traveled from Okinawa to Tokyo on behalf of the Ministry of Education in Japan. At the demonstration, Gichin impressed Jigoro Kano (the father of Judo) and Hakudo Nakayama (Kendo Master) so ended up staying in Tokyo to introduce Karate to the major universities of Japan. At age 55 in year 1923, Gichin had very few students and lived in poverty saying "To pay for the tiny room where I slept, I took on odd jobs at the dormitory: watchman, caretaker, gardener, and even room sweeper."

At the close of World War II in 1945, U.S. General Douglas MacArthur banned the teaching of Judo and Kendo in Japan. Fortunately for Karate, Professor Ohama asked the U.S. Occupational Force to classify Karate as physical education not a martial art, which allowed Gichin to teach martial artists from other disciplines looking for permitted "martial arts" such as Karate. Gichin's biggest contribution was when he sent Karate instructors to the United States in the 1950s per request of United States citizens who learned basic techniques from returning American soldiers.

Famous karateka are James Caan, Madonna, Elvis Presley, Sean Connery (James Bond), D'Brickashaw Ferguson (NFL Athlete), James Johnson (NBA Player), Steven Ho (stuntman), Chuck Norris, Jean-Claude Van Damme, Georges St-Pierre (UFC Fighter), Taylor Lautner ("Twilight" show), and Wesley Snipes. Best films featuring karate are "Blood Sport" featuring Jean-Claude Van Damme and "The Karate Kid" featuring Noriyuki Morita. You can learn more about karate in Gichin Funakoshi's books titled "Karate-do kyohan" and "Karate-do: my way of life."

Gichin lays out "The Twenty Guiding Principles of Karate." The principles are: training begins and ends with bowing, there is no first strike in karate, Karate stands on the side of justice, First know yourself then know others, Mentality over technique, The heart must be set free, Calamity springs from carelessness, Karate goes beyond the dojo, Karate is a lifelong pursuit, Apply the way of karate to all things - therein lies its beauty, Karate is like boiling water where water returns to its tepid without heat, Do not think of winning and instead think of not losing, Make adjustments according to your opponent, The outcome of a battle depends on how one handles emptiness and fullness, Think of hands and feet as swords, You face a million enemies when you step beyond your own gate, Formal stances are for beginners - one stands naturally, Perform prescribed sets of techniques exactly - actual combat is another matter, Do not forget the employment of withdrawal of power/the extension or contraction of the body/the swift or leisurely application of technique, and Be constantly mindful, diligent, and resourceful, in your pursuit of the Way.

MUAY THAI - NAI KHANOMTOM 1767

Known as the "Art of Eight Limbs," Muay Thai uses the fists, elbows, feet, and shins. Many UFC fighters today use Muay Thai's low shin kicks, flying knees, back fists, and reverse elbows in competition. Legendary Muay Thai fighters are Samart Payakaroon (Muhammed Ali of Muay Thai),

Tony Jaa, Sagat Petchyindee (Sagat in "Street Fighter" game), Saenchai, Pud Pad Noy Worawoot (Golden Leg), Somrak Kamsing (Olympic Gold Medalist), Apidej Sit-Hirun, Buakaw Banchamek, and Ryan Gosling ("Only God Forgives" movie). Best films displaying Muay Thai are "Ong Bak" featuring Tony Jaa and "Kickboxer" featuring Jean-Claude van Damme.

At age 43, actor Idris Elba trained 12 months for 1 professional Muay Thai fight in his documentary "Idris Elba: Fighter." Idris said his motivation for training was "It was part of being a man. Facing up to another man is the ultimate test. Are you going to back down or are you going to face the fear? Everyone thinks they're hard. When push comes to shove, what are you going to do? Do you have the physical and mental strength to protect yourself?"

In 1238, the first Thai army was created in the northern city of Sukhothai to protect the government and its people. With constant threat of war, men practiced Muay Thai for self-defense, exercise, and discipline. Muay Thai became popular where high-class and royalty were required to practice Muay Thai as good warriors made brave leaders.

In 1767, Thailand was ransacked by Lord Mangra's Burmese army. To celebrate the Burmese victory, Lord Mangra threw a festival ordering Thai prisoners to fight the best Burmese fighters. Nai Khanom Tom "Father of Muay Thai" defeated 10 consecutive elite Burmese fighters. Impressed, Lord Mangra said to Nai "Every part of the Siamese is blessed with venom. Even with his bare hands, he can defeat ten opponents. But his Lord was incompetent and lost the country to the enemy" and rewarded Nai freedom and Burmese women as wives. Nai Khanom Tom returned to Thailand as a hero and spent the rest of his life teaching Muay Thai. Nai is remembered every year on March 17 as the greatest Muay Thai fighter in history.

JUDO - KANO JIGORO 1882

At age 14, Kanō Jigorō started to train judo when he experienced bullying at school. Judo known as the "gentle way" was created as a physical, mental, and moral discipline that involves throwing an opponent to the ground to defeat them with a pinning technique. Judo fighters don't have to depend on pure strength against bigger opponents.

Famous judoka are Vladimir Putin (Russian President), Theodore Roosevelt (U.S. President), Prince Albert of Monaco, Mick Jagger, Naomi Watts, Ben Campbell (U.S. Senator for Colorado), William Hague (leader of Conservative Party in the UK), Pierre Trudeau (former Prime Minister of Canada, Justin Trudeau's father), and Yoshitsugu Yamashita (taught U.S.

President Theodore Roosevelt). To get a taste of Judo, you can watch Vladimir Putin's film titled "Let's Learn Judo with Vladimir Putin."

During 1910 in the United Kingdom when women were fighting for the right to vote, police officers and men with a minimum height of 5 ft 10 inches or 178cm, physically abused women. With most women having average height of 4ft 11 inch or 150cm, Edith Garrud was inspired about Judo's capability to help smaller people defeat larger opponents so taught Judo to the Women's Social and Political Union (WSPU). "Health and Strength" magazine printed a satirical article called "Jiu-jitsuffragettes." This amazing story of strong British women using judo martial arts for self defense is captured in the movie "Suffragette."

BRAZILIAN JIU-JITSU - HELIO GRACIE 1929

Brazilian jiu-jitsu's (BJJ) is based on the concept that a smaller and weaker person can defeat a stronger and heavier opponent by using leverage to take the fight to the ground where you defeat the opponent with joint locks and chokeholds. BJJ's techniques comes from Judo when Judo founder Kano Jigoro sent his top 5 students overseas to spread the art.

Famous Brazilian jiu-jitsu practitioners are Keanu Reeves (Matrix, John Wick), Demi Lovato (singer), Henry Cavill (Superman), Scarlett Johansson (Black Widow in "Iron Man"), Margot Robbie ("Suicide Squad" movie), Tom Hardy (Mad Max), Ashton Kutcher, Vince Vaughn, Guy Ritchie (movie director), Kelly Slater (surfer), Anthony Bourdain, Jim Carrey, Nicholas Cage, Mel Gibson, Steve Irwin, and Ed O'Neill. Best films featuring Brazilian jiu-jitsu are "Red Belt" featuring Chiwetel Ejiofor and "Warrior" featuring Tom Hardy. You can learn more about BJJ by books written by Helio Gracie himself titled "Gracie Jiu-Jitsu: The Master Text" and "Gracie Submission Essentials: Grandmaster and Master Secrets of Finishing a Fight."

With mixed martial arts popularity, UFC President Dana White, the Gracie Family, and Bruce Lee's training partner Dan Inosanto all credit Bruce Lee as the "Father of Mixed Martial Arts who was 50 years ahead of his time."

Born in 1902, Carlos Gracie was aggressive getting in fights and being expelled from schools. In 1917 when Carlos was 15 years old, his father Gastao took him to a professional wrestling challenge hosted in his circus at the Da Paz Theatre in Brazil. After Carlos Gracie watched a demonstration where Judoka Mitsuyo Maeda defeats a bigger man, Maeda accepted Carlos as a student. Beginning in 1929, Hélio Gracie, who learned BJJ from his brother Carlos, developed Gracie Jiu Jitsu as an adaptation from judo.

The Gracie violence re-emerged with Carlos Gracie and the Gracie Brothers including Hélio attacked Carlos' 1931 opponent Manoel Rufino dos Santos where the Gracie family knocked out Rufino with a steel box so Carlos could dislocate Rufino's shoulder with an armlock. This despicable incident resulted in a career-ending injury to Rufino and the brothers serving 2.5 years in prison for assault.

As the face of BJJ, the Gracie family must promote self defense and humility in defeat instead of assaulting winners as sore losers. When Carlos Gracie died, he passed BJJ down to his 21 children, 106 grandchildren, and 128 great-grandchildren.

KRAV MAGA - IMI LICHTENFELD 1930

Krav Maga is a military self-defense system developed for the Israel Defense Forces (IDF) influenced by boxing, wrestling, Aikido, judo, and karate. The fighting system was formed from Imi's street-fighting experience defending his Jewish quarter against fascist groups in Bratislava, Czechoslovakia during the 1930s. Asian martial arts influence on Krav Maga came when Imi's top student Eli Avikzar incorporating aikido elements in 1971 and using Judo's belt ranking system.

Imi Lichtenfeld, the founder of Krav Maga, was born in 1910. His father Samuel was a Chief Detective in Bratislava who trained officers in self-defense and also trained Imi. In the 1930s, fascist and anti-Semitic groups started to attack Bratislava's Jewish community. Within the next 10 years, Imi's countless fights against the anti-Semitic thugs to protect his Jewish community helped him craft the Krav Maga self-defense system against hand and weapon attacks. In 1940, Imi boarded the last immigrant ship to Israel in escaping the Nazis. In 1944, General Itzchak Sadeh of the Hagana resistance force called Imi to train the Israel Defense Forces (IDF) military organization in physical fitness, swimming, attacking with a knife, and defending against knife attacks. After retiring from military duty, Imi adapted Krav Maga to civilian needs where man or woman, boy or girl, or young or old people can learn fast. Today in Israel, Krav Maga is taught at schools, universities, businesses, and in community centers.

Imi Lichtenfeld (the Father of Krav Maga) from his book "Krav Maga" famously says "Everyone wants to be in someone else's place: At the circus a young, muscular gymnast performs acrobatic feats on the trapeze, while in the audience below, in the most expensive seat, sits a rich, fat businessman with a cigar between his lips and a stunning girl on his arm. The businessman says to himself: "I would give all I have in order to be like him, young, athletics, without a care in the world," and the acrobat, who sees him from high up on the trapeze, thinks: "I wish I could be in his place, a rich man with such a beautiful woman, who can afford the most expensive seat at the circus and watch a young, poor, unfortunate guy like me endanger his life for a few cents." Imi stresses that both health and wealth are important.

Celebrity Krav Maga practitioners are Gal Gadot (Wonder Woman), Brad Pitt, Angelina Jolie ("Tomb Raider" movie), Daniel Craig (James Bond), Jennifer Lopez ("Enough" movie), Tom Cruise (Mission Impossible), Hilary Swank ("Million Dollar Baby" movie), Jessica Chastain ("The Debt" movie), Sean Penn ("The Gunman" movie), and Leonardo Dicaprio ("Blood Diamond" movie). Best movies featuring Krav Maga are "The Debt" featuring Jessica Chastain, "Salt" featuring Angelina Jolie, "Enough" featuring Jennifer Lopez, "Collateral" featuring Tom Cruise, and "Casino Royale" featuring Daniel Craig. You can learn more about Krav Maga by reading "Krav Maga: How to Defend Yourself Against Armed Assault" by Imi Lichtenfeld and "Complete Krav Maga: The Ultimate Guide to Over 250 Self-Defense and Combative Techniques" by Darren Levine.

Imi's most famous sayings from his "Krav Maga" book are "Before beginning to court a woman, you would better know who her father is, who her brothers are, and sometimes even who her boyfriend is" and "Sometimes a man turns his head to look at a woman and it changes his entire life, and sometimes he does not turn his head and that too changes his life."

TAE KWON DO - JHOON RHEE 1950

Beginning in 1945 after the end of World War II, new martial arts schools called kwans opened in Seoul by Korean martial artists with experience in Japanese, Chinese and Korean martial arts. A heavy emphasis was placed on kicking as using legs in combat gave them an edge over fighting styles that focus on punching. Taekwondo became popular with civilians when the South Korean military used Taekwondo in their martial arts training.

Celebrity Taekwondo practitioners are President Barack Obama, Bas Rutten (UFC Fighter), Sarah Michelle Gellar ("Buffer the Vampire Slayer" show), Jessica Alba, Evan Rachel Wood ("Westworld" show), Michael Imperioli (Sopranos), Joe Rogan ("Fear Factor" host), Kylie Minogue, Rick Yune, and Katheryn Winnick. The best films featuring Taekwondo are "When Taekwondo Strikes" featuring Jhoon Rhee, "Best of the Best" featuring Tommy Lee, and "The City of Violence" featuring Ryoo Seung-wan. You can read more about Taekwondo in Jhoon Rhee's form books, "Ultimate Flexibility: A Complete Guide to Stretching for Martial Arts" by Sang H. Kim, and "Complete Taekwondo Poomsae: The Official Tangeuk, Palgwae, and Black Belt Forms of Taekwondo" by Sang H. Kim.

Although South Korean army general Choi Hong Hi is credited with creating Taekwondo, Hi's student Jhoon Rhee is known as the "Father of American Taekwondo" for spreading martial arts in the United States in the 1950s.

Born in 1932 during the Japanese occupation of Korea, Jhoon broke his thigh bone at age 3 when he was accidentally dropped by his 7-year-old sister. Because of the accident, Rhee's family believed he would never be athletic. Jhoon says "I was the smallest, weakest, most uncoordinated kid in school...when I was 6, a 5-year-old girl beat me up...I was always last in track races." Determined to prove critics wrong about his size and speed, he wanted to learn martial arts but couldn't as Japanese colonial rule banned all martial arts practices similar to what happened with Karate's ban. Fortunately at age 13 in year 1945, Korea gained independence from Japanese rule so the ban on martial arts teaching was lifted - allowing Jhoon to study with Grandmaster Won Kook Lee in Seoul 2 years later at age 15.

In a self-defense fight against a bully in the 11th grade in front of his classmates, Jhoon countered the bully's punch by punching the boy in the eye and kicking him in the throat. The "stand up to the bully" fight garnered respect for Jhoon as a confident person despite his small size.

Inspired by American soldiers who helped push the North Korean communists out of South Korea, Jhoon wanted to repay his gratitude with a military stint in America and then was sponsored by an elderly couple to stay in the United States. Jhoon says "America has really helped Korea, and I am so grateful for this...more than 34,000 young Americans sacrificed their lives for a country they never heard of and people they never met...then the Americans helped rebuild Korea's economy into what it is today."

In 1962 at age 30, Jhoon opened his first Taekwondo studio in Washington D.C. using marketing tactics such as writing letters to ambassadors serving in D.C. stressing Taekwondo can help their children achieve A's and B's in school, running ads in the sports section of the Washington Post, and producing a TV commercial ad featuring his daughter saying the anti-bullying slogan "Nobody Bothers Me" followed by his son saying "Nobody bothers me, either."

Jhoon's impact on Capitol Hill came in 1965 when he read the news of Rep. James Cleveland of New Hampshire being mugged so Jhoon called

Cleveland's office about teaching Rep. Cleveland martial arts. Cleveland appreciated the offer so much that he asked his Capitol Hill colleagues if they were interested in martial arts that led to the U.S. Congressional Tae Kwon Do Club. Since then, Jhoon has trained over 350 members of Congress including President Lyndon Johnson, President George H.W. Bush, Vice President Joe Biden, Speaker Newt Gingrich (R-Georgia), Rep. Bob Livingston (R-Louisiana), Rep. Jesse Jackson Jr. (D-Illinois), Rep. Carolyn Maloney (D-New York), and Rep. Duncan Hunter (R-California).

In 1964, Jhoon met Bruce Lee at a martial arts tournament in Long Beach, California where the two became great friends with Bruce Lee teaching Jhoon his most powerful move "the one-inch punch" and Jhoon showing Bruce flashy powerful kicks. Wanting to show Taekwondo to the world similar to Bruce Lee did with Chinese martial arts, Bruce helped Jhoon in 1972 with a Taekwondo movie starring Jhoon. Unfortunately, Bruce Lee died before the release of Jhoon's movie. Heartbroken, Jhoon said "I mourned not only the loss of my friend, but the loss to the world of martial arts as Bruce would have continued to make invaluable contributions to the philosophy so I was satisfied when I passed on Bruce Lee's legacy to Muhammad Ali - teaching him the "Accupunch" to defeat Joe Frazier and Richard Dunn."

Jhoon's goal was to live until 136 like a supercentenarian but he passed away in year 2018 at age 86. At his funeral, U.S. Representative Nick Smith praised Jhoon's teachings as "a philosophy grounded in the principles of the martial arts, but applicable to everyone. It calls for people to build confidence through knowledge in the mind, honesty in the heart, and strength in the body, and then to lead by example."

Today, all Taekwondo practitioners abide by Choi Hong Hi's five tenets of: I shall observe the tenets (courtesy, integrity, perseverance, self-control, indomitable spirit) of taekwondo, I shall respect the instructor and seniors, I shall never misuse taekwondo, I shall be a champion of freedom and justice, I shall build a more peaceful world.

JEET KUNE DO - BRUCE LEE 1967

Born in 1940, Bruce Lee died at the early age of 32 years old. His impact as a martial artist and actor inspired the world especially Asian and African American communities as Bruce Lee was the first famous person of color to be featured as a protagonist. Bruce proved that Asian men can be strong and sexy. For example, the Wu-Tang Clan rap group says Bruce Lee inspired them to pursue martial arts. Quentin Tarantino had Uma Thurman in

Bruce Lee's signature yellow costume in "Kill Bill." Even the State of New York banned nunchucks, popularized by Bruce Lee's "Enter the Dragon" movie, since 1974 until U.S. District Judge Pamela Chen declared New York's ban as unconstitutional since the possession of a martial arts weapon is protected under the Second Amendment. Per Matthew Polly, author of "Bruce Lee: A Life," "Bruce Lee had bigger goals than just being a movie and martial arts star as he modeled his career after Clint Eastwood. He went to Hollywood in the same way Eastwood went to Italy to make a few cheap movies to prove his bankability to Hollywood. He would've acted for a couple more decades in various films and then gone behind the camera as a director."

Celebrity Jeet Kune Do practitioners are Kobe Bryant ("Black Mamba" mentality as an NBA player), Uma Thurman ("Kill Bill" movie), Dan Inosanto (Bruce Lee's training partner), Kareem Abdul Jabbar (Bruce Lee Student, NBA star, "Game of Death" film), Michael Jackson, Anderson Silva (UFC Fighter), Phil Mickelson, Steve McQueen (Bruce Lee Student, Hollywood rival and friend of Bruce Lee), James Coburn (Bruce Lee Student), Robert F Diggs (Wu Tang Clan), Glenn Danzig, Criss Angel, Sharon Tate (Bruce Lee Student, murdered by members of Manson Family), James Garner (Bruce Lee Student, "Marlowe" movie), George Lazenby (Bruce Lee Student, "James Bond" film), and Taky Kimura (Bruce Lee's top student and best man at Bruce Lee's wedding).

The best depiction of Jeet Kune Do is "The Legend of Bruce Lee" starring Danny Chan which is a television series based on the life of Bruce Lee. You can read more about Jeet Kune Do in Bruce Lee's "The Tao of Jeet Kune Do," "Bruce Lee Striking Thoughts: Bruce Lee's Wisdom for Daily Living," and "Bruce Lee: The Art of Expressing the Human Body." Also read Teri Tom's "The Straight Lead: The Core of Bruce Lee's Jun Fan Jeet Kune Do" and Matthew Polly's "Bruce Lee: A Life."

In 1940, Bruce Lee was born in San Francisco to father Lee Hoi-chuen who was a famous Hong Kong actor in the United States for an acting residency and to mother Grace Ho who was of Eurasian ancestry (Bruce was a quarter English, an eighth Dutch-Jewish and five-eighths Chinese) and the half-niece of Robert Ho-tung (one of the wealthiest and influential person in Hong Kong). As such, Bruce Lee grew up in an affluent and privileged childhood.

Being Eurasian or not fully 100% Chinese blood was difficult for Bruce Lee as he faced racism from Americans when he was in the United States and from Chinese in Hong Kong. Hong Kong waited 32 years after Bruce Lee's death to dedicate a statue to him in 2005. When people asked

Bruce if he was American or Chinese, he would say "I think of myself as a human being first." Studying Wing Chun martial arts under the famous Ip man became difficult when his peers refused to be in the same class as a Eurasian as the Chinese were generally against teaching martial arts to non-Asians so Ip Man had to teach Bruce Lee privately. Being Eurasian helped Bruce Lee be open to teaching non-Asians as he was mixed race. Bruce Lee's first martial arts student was African American Jesse Glover who couldn't find any martial arts teachers willing to take a black student. Bruce openly worked with African Americans in Hollywood such as NBA superstar Kareem Abdul-Jabbar in the movie "Game of Death."

Due to Bruce Lee's strong and sexy body, men wanted to be Bruce and women wanted to be with Bruce. Bruce Lee taught martial arts to actors James Coburn and Steve McQueen, inspired elite athletes like basketball player Kobe Bryant to derive his killer "Mamba Mentality" from Bruce Lee, gave rise to mixed martial arts tournaments with UFC President Dana White saying Bruce Lee is the "Father of MMA," and instructed World Karate Champions Chuck Norris, Joe Lewis, and Mike Stone.

Bruce Lee found love in 1964 when he married his college classmate and martial arts student Linda Emery. However, Bruce Lee came from two cultures which didn't believe in monogamy with Hong Kong in the 1950s where Bruce's grandfather had 13 concubines and during the 1960s "Free Love" era in America. As such, Bruce had love affairs with several women during his marriage such as Sharon Farrell who said "Bruce took me to the moon and back as he was so knowledgeable about a woman's body," both Nara Miao and Betty Ting Pei from "Way of the Dragon" film, and Thordis Brandt who was attracted to Bruce for his amazing cha-cha dancing.

What made Bruce different from martial arts founders was that he was a bully. In his youth, Bruce formed a gang of troublemakers and got expelled from his Catholic school for pulling a knife on a gym instructor. Bullying became dangerous in the spring of 1959 when Bruce beat the son of a feared triad family with the police warning his father that there was a contract out for Bruce's life. Concerned, Bruce's father sent him to live with his sister in San Francisco, United States.

In Oakland's Chinatown in 1964, Bruce had a controversial private martial arts match with Wong Jack Man who the Chinese community sent to discipline Bruce for teaching martial arts to non-Asians. If Bruce lost, he would have to close his school. Fortunately, Bruce defeated Wong Jack Man in three minutes and continued teaching to people of all races.

3 years later in 1967, Bruce Lee founded Jeet Kune Do martial arts

mainly thru his fight with Wong Jack Man that lasted too long and wasted energy. So Bruce developed a system with an emphasis on practicality, flexibility, speed, and efficiency. Bruce felt that many martial artists of his time did not spend enough time on physical conditioning so he started weight training for muscle mass without losing speed or flexibility, running for endurance, jumping rope for footwork and agility, stretching for flexibility, and ate healthy such as drinking raw hamburger meat smoothies for protein.

Jeet Kune Do favors formlessness as Bruce Lee famously says "Empty your mind, be formless, shapeless, like water. If you put water into a cup, it becomes the cup. You put water into a bottle and it becomes the bottle. You put it in a teapot it becomes the teapot...Be water, my friend." For fighting technique, Jeet Kune Do uses an oblique leg kick to block an attacker's potential kick, forearm blocks against hook punches, a non-telegraphed punch that you initiate without any forewarning such as tensing your shoulders or moving your foot (Muhammad Ali learned this punch from Bruce Lee thru Jhoon Rhee), stop-hitting opponents when they're trying to get within striking distance, and simultaneous parry with punching so you utilize the opponent's energy against them by creating an imbalance.

In 1969, Bruce Lee worked with screenwriter Stirling Silliphant and actor James Coburn on a script for a film called "The Silent Flute" facing the difficulty that Hollywood didn't believe that American audiences would accept an Asian hero. Disappointed with Hollywood, Producer Fred Weintraub advised Bruce to make successful films in Hong Kong to impress Hollywood which Bruce did with "The Big Boss" in 1971, "Fist of Fury" in 1972, and "Way of the Dragon" with Chuck Norris in 1972.

Now with Hollywood's attention, Bruce Lee died six days before the release of "Enter the Dragon" in 1973. According to press, Bruce was experiencing a headache when he was rehearsing "The Game of Death" script in Betty Ting's apartment so Betty gave Bruce a tablet of Equagesic - an aspirin-based drug that she often used herself. Bruce didn't wake up for a dinner appointment with Golden Harvest owner Raymond Chow. There are many takes on Bruce's death with Raymond Chow saying Bruce died from an allergic reaction to the meprobamate ingredient in the Equagesic pill, Chuck Norris saying Bruce died from a mixing of Equagesic and the muscle-relaxant medication he took for a ruptured disc in his back, and others saying the Chinese triads came after Bruce for bullying children of Mafia bosses and teaching martial arts to non-Asian people. In addition to suffering from pain killers, autopsies reveal that Bruce Lee suffered from an "Asian flush" enzyme deficiency from alcohol and smoking too much marijuana as "Enter the

Dragon" costar Bob Wall says "Bruce would require two weed brownies before he would calm down into a normal person."

Bruce Lee's death at such a young age was devastating for the progression of featuring Asian stars in Hollywood that we still don't see today. Buried in Seattle, Bruce's pallbearers were Taky Kimura (Bruce Lee's best friend and certified Jeet Kune Do instructor), Steve McQueen (Bruce Lee student who introduced Bruce to marijuana), James Coburn (Bruce Lee student who would have starred together in "The Silent Flute" movie), Chuck Norris ("Way of the Dragon" costar), George Lazenby (credited Bruce Lee for reviving his career as "James Bond"), Dan Inosanto (Bruce Lee's training partner and certified Jeet Kune Do instructor), Peter Chin (Bruce Lee's student), and Robert Lee (Bruce's brother).

JUSTHUYNH FITNESS - FRANCIS HUYNH 2016

Born in 1988, the year of the Dragon, I was born in Maine to Vietnamese parents who came over to the United States as boat people to save their income from blue collar jobs so my brother and I could achieve the American Dream thru education.

Having overcome obesity, racism, bullying, and discrimination thru martial arts, my mission, just like the founders of Shaolin, Karate, Muay Thai, Krav Maga, and Taekwondo did to overcome bullying and racism, is to empower the 2 billion overweight people worldwide thru martial arts via online training and thousands of studios in major cities around the world.

JustHuynh Fitness' "Ageless Athletic Assassin" philosophy emphasizes the need to adopt healthy habits to age gracefully, train cardio to stay in terrific shape, and practice martial arts for self defense. By committing to our philosophy, you will be able to thrive personally with a significant other, academically in intelligence, athletically, and professionally at work.

Per the FBI Crime Clock, an assault occurs every 26.3 seconds. Per RAINN (Rape, Abuse, & Incest National Network), Americans are sexually assaulted every 98 seconds. There was a time when governments banned the teaching of Karate and Taekwondo due to fear that martial artists could overthrow the government, but fortunately the majority of countries allow the practice of martial arts and I hope you take advantage of this.

Fitness should be a healthy habit just like brushing your teeth, Anyone can setup a free-standing kicking bag in their home, college dorm room, office, small business, public place, and gym where JustHuynh Fitness' martial arts and power athletics can be practiced.

CHAPTER 6

JustHuynh Fitness Origins

No citizen has a right to be an amateur in the matter of physical training...what a disgrace it is for a man to grow old without ever seeing the beauty and strength of which his body is capable

- Socrates

VIETNAM WAR POW - FRANCIS OF ASSISI

My father served as a lieutenant in the South Vietnamese Army commanding hundreds of soldiers. The North Vietnamese's ability to wear down the American soldier's will to fight and ultimate retreat is one of the most shocking feats in warfare history. As such my father along with 300,000 other Vietnamese men associated with the South Vietnamese government (former military officers, government workers and South Vietnam supporters) became prisoners of war who were sent to re-education camp where many endured torture, starvation, and disease while being forced to perform hard labor such as mine field sweeping. My father mentioned that prisoners were organized into work units who competed against each other in hard labor. Teams who lost hard labor competitions were sent to confinement in 4 feet high by 4 feet wide Conex boxes where prisoners were allowed one bowl of rice and a cup of water a day. Many of my father's compatriots couldn't handle re-education so spoke out during class. They were immediately pulled outside class, shot, and never seen again. Knowing North Vietnam's zero tolerance policy and opportunity to return home after a couple years of being an abiding prisoner, my father survived reeducation camp and returned home to Da Nang and then resettled in Saigon.

All boat people had a 50% chance of being killed in open water by the North Vietnamese - 350,000 of 700,000 boat people died in open water by getting shot at or raped, robbed, and killed by Thai pirates. When captured, women were raped in front of their husbands before being thrown overboard with their children and grandparents, whereas physically able men were used for slave labor until they starved to death. When my father escaped one night in Soc Trang via boat by exchanging gold for 2 4-person boats, my father told his dad that if my grandfather did not hear back from my dad within a year that meant my dad died in a failed attempt to freedom. After securing the 2 4-person boats for my uncle, two teenage cousin males, and my father's relative's family of four thru secret verbal code, they sailed to a 90-person boat that aggregated smaller boats in 1 day. If my Father had been caught by the North Vietnamese Army, he would have been shot in the head for not abiding by his re-education. It took 3 days to sail from the 90-person boat location to Bidong Island in Malaysia. For protection, my dad and a former South Vietnamese soldier each held a hand grenade in case they encountered Thai Pirates. Fortunately, my father did not encounter Thai Pirates but it was dangerous at the island's entrance where native Malaysians threw glass at the boat people due to jealousy that Vietnamese refugees would get new life as immigrants to the United States thru the United Nations help.

Bidong Island, a one square kilometer area in Malaysia where boat people from Vietnam sailed to, was the most heavily populated place on Earth where 40,000 boat people refugees awaited for resettlement by the United Nations in 1979. The Malaysian government threatened to kill all Vietnamese refugees until U.S. President Jimmy Carter agreed to accept 14,000 Vietnamese refugees a month as immigrants. Living conditions were terrible where water was rationed at one gallon per day per person and medicine was in short supply for tropical diseases. By the time Bidong camp closed in 1991, over 250,000 Vietnamese had stayed before being resettled to the United States, Canada, Australia, or France. After 9 months living on the island, my father and mother were very fortunate to have been sponsored by Priest Father Donald Gilbert from Lewiston, Maine who we visited every Christmas until his passing when I was in middle school.

Grateful for life in America, my dad gave Priest Father Donald Gilbert the liberty of choosing my brother and I's English first names. I was named Francis, similar to current Pope Francis, after Francis of Assisi because Father Gilbert wanted me to "never forget the poor" since my parents came over with nothing as boat people from Vietnam. If I become successful, Father Gilbert's wish is for me to help the less fortunate achieve success.

Settling in Maine, which is the whitest state in America where 95% of the 1 million population is white and only 1% is Asian, my mom served the small Vietnamese community by making monthly 4 hour long round-trips to Boston to rent dubbed over Chinese TV series on videotape for the Vietnamese community in Portland, Maine to watch as the 1980s and 1990s were an era before online streaming killed videotapes and DVDs. My mom did this for fun as a way to help families enjoy their free time away from work. Her main job has been working as a press launder at minimum wage. As a Lieutenant prisoner of war for the South Vietnamese who survived re-education camp before escaping on boat to Malaysia and then sponsorship to the United States, my father is the highest ranking South Vietnamese soldier in Maine. His leadership helps people recover from post traumatic stress disorder (PTSD) and integrate into white America as a minority. My dad works in a minimum wage job installing wafers into semiconductor chips - saving his earning for my brother and I to obtain a 4-year college degree from Bowdoin College - proving that the American Dream can be achieved by people who come to America with nothing and rise up thru education.

For PTSD, over 3 million families are still living with the effects of Agent Orange where the United States Army sprayed over 13 million gallons of the deadly herbicide chemical dioxin, produced by Monsanto and Dow Chemical, on Vietnam from 1961 to 1971 that caused serious health issues such as cancer, birth defects to 500,000 children, rashes, spina bifida, cleft palettes, a decrease in immunity, disorders in the endocrine system, reproduction disorders, and severe psychological and neurological problems.

When new families immigrate to Maine, my father is the first person Vietnamese call to help obtain their two most important documents: U.S. Passport and Driver's License. A U.S. Passport helps Vietnamese travel freely outside the United States and a driver's license helps people commute on their own. Many Vietnamese Americans make a living in the service industry with pho restaurants, nail salons, hardwood flooring, and car maintenance.

Raising future first generation college graduates as a minority in the 1980s was not easy especially with my mother's highest education being 7th grade as she had to care for family and sell dishes during the Vietnam War and my dad's English proficiency at a basic level. Although my parents couldn't help me with English homework or tutor me in the school subjects, my mom provided my brother and I great care and encouragement that education is the key to success. If we give our best effort in grade school to graduate in the top of our high school class, we can get admitted into one of the best colleges in America (Bowdoin College undergrad, Columbia Engineering (brother) and Vanderbilt MBA (me)) in order to land lucrative six figure careers thru merit. This was not easy as I spoke broken English until the 6th grade, having to be pulled out of the classroom once a day to improve my English. It didn't help that I was bullied for being skinny, weak, dumb, shy, and Asian. I tried my best to learn English from watching my favorite TV Show "Dragon Ball Z" and to learn my native language Vietnamese by watching the dubbed over

Chinese movies such as "Journey to the West - featuring Monkey King." With no nearby family for help, my dad has worked the night shift from 6PM to 6AM to alternate shifts watching over my brother and I with my mom who worked from 7AM to 4PM. My Father was the motivator to ensure we were excelling in academics and leadership activities like track, student government, math team, and music.

MARTIAL ARTS LIFE CHANGER

With experience in martial arts in the South Vietnamese army and noticing the lower confidence I was exhibiting from bullying and racism, one of the best gifts was when my father enrolled my brother and I in karate for 3 years with Master Tony Fournier in Portland Maine beginning in the 6th grade that helped us with confidence, self defense against bullying, enhanced cognitive function to achieve high grades for admission into elite colleges in America, and improved athleticism to captain the track teams. Aside from self defense, martial arts is a philosophy in itself that taught us discipline, respect, confidence, leadership, teamwork, and humbleness to be a great human being.

HIGH SCHOOL TRACK CAPTAIN

As a first generation Asian American family learning to enjoy life in Maine, my mom and dad didn't have the knowledge or connections about youth sports such as soccer, basketball, or baseball where star student athletes can get college paid for thru athletic scholarships.

We were fortunate to have been welcomed by legendary South Portland High School indoor and outdoor track coaches Paul Brogan and John Chapin. What's great about track is that everyone is accepted on the team. Coming in as the shortest athlete on the team at 5 feet 2 inches and overweight, both coaches helped me become a fit athlete and leader. In high school, I challenged myself in the 55 meter hurdle race where I had to jump over four 3 feet high hurdles in under 7 seconds. This was one of the toughest challenges in my life as I'm only 5 feet 2 inches tall.

Over the four years in high school, my coaches named me as one of the four high school track captains to lead the team of seventy track athletes recognizing my dedication to high intensity interval training and leadership ability to help transform students from slow to fast.

COLLEGE SERVICE EXPERIENCE

Dunkin Donuts was my first job making $7 an hour during the college summers where I worked the morning shift and learned how to deliver fast and accurate orders for caffeine needy customers. I also sold Cutco Cutlery performing 1-hour presentations to over 200 households and developed the ability to understand customer pain points where sharper and longer-lasting knives provided for a better cooking experience.

Interning for Morgan Stanley Smith Barney for $10 an hour one summer, I learned that private wealth managers provide the best service to high net-worth clients by keeping short-term and long-term financial goals just like one would for their health such as a weight target or race time.

HEALTH IS WEALTH

My four years as a management consultant for PricewaterhouseCoopers (PwC) is a world class organization that JustHuynh Fitness strives for. Just like all Fortune 500 and private companies hire PwC to audit their financials or provide strategy consulting, companies also have to ensure their employees are physically fit to thrive at work. Travelling the world, it was amazing to see PwC dominate the skylines of major cities. JustHuynh Fitness' goal is to be the "third place" globally where people can come to improve their health so they can enjoy their wealth.

WORLD CLASS PREMIUM EXPERIENCE

At Samsung, I learned what it takes to be the 4th most valuable brand in the world by providing customers with premium products and experiences. Samsung's mission is to "Inspire the world with our innovative technologies, products, and design that enrich people's lives and contribute to social prosperity by creating a new future." JustHuynh Fitness' mission is to provide the fastest and safest martial arts and power athletics training for the over 2 billion overweight people worldwide to be strong, sexy, and smart.

SUPER AGENTS OF JUSTICE

Having received an offer with the FBI, one of the most respected law enforcement agencies in the world, candidates must be mentally (at least two years of professional full-time experience) and physically (maintain a high level of fitness by passing the FBI Fitness Test) strong. To deliver the best training, JustHuynh Fitness' instructors have at least two years of martial arts training while also maintaining a high fitness level by scoring at least 70 points in all events (hex-bar deadlift, power throw, release pushups, sprint/drag/carry, leg tuck, and 2 mile run) of the Army Combat Fitness Test.

ROCKSTAR GLOBAL INFLUENCE

In 2018 my wife and I attended our first in-person music concert - choosing Taylor Swift's "Reputation" stadium tour in Boston at Gillette Stadium. It was inspiring to see the impact Taylor has made in people's lives as she performed 53 shows generating $345.7 million in ticket sales to over 3 million fans - which is the highest grossing tour ever.

As two of the 60,000 fans in attendance, it was inspiring to see mostly females sing from the bottom of their hearts as they relate to Taylor's lyrics about love and heartbreak with men. During JustHuynh Fitness' 45-minute classes, we have upbeat music to get you energized. Like Taylor connecting with audiences from all over the world thru music about love, JustHuynh Fitness aims to positively change people's lives thru martial arts.

BOWDOIN COMMON GOOD - MIND

Bowdoin College in my home state of Maine seeks students who are "bright and have a willingness to take intellectual risks as well as a commitment to the Common Good." Former Bowdoin President Joseph McKeen described the "Common Good" commitment as "It ought always to be remembered, that literary institutions are founded and endowed for the common good, and not for the private advantage of those who resort to them for education. It is not that they may be enabled to pass through life in an easy or reputable manner, but that their mental powers may be cultivated and improved for the benefit of society."

At JustHuynh Fitness, we provide members the best martial arts and power athletics so they can use their mental and physical strength to improve society. Their physical powers should only be used for self defense and never to harm good human beings.

VANDERBILT COMMODORE CREED - BODY

Spending two years in Nashville to obtain my MBA at Vanderbilt gave rise to JustHuynh Fitness' mission to boost people's confidence and self defense thru martial arts. As the fittest and brightest university in the world, Vanderbilt athletes abide to the "Commodore Creed" below:

Never underestimate your opponent.

Work on your weaknesses until they become your strong points.

Remember that a great effort is usually the result of a great attitude.

Dedicate yourself to a mighty purpose.

Win with humility, lose with grace.

Ignore those who discourage you.

Work to improve your moral and spiritual strengths as well as your physical ones.

Remember that how you conduct yourself off the field is just important as how you conduct yourself on the field.

Talent is God given - be humble.

Fame is man given - be thankful.

Conceit is self given - be careful.

Don't ask to be deprived of tension and discipline - those are tools that shape success.

Do what has to be done, when it has to be done, and as well as it can be done.

Remember that when you are not working to improve, your competition is.

Always give you best.

Practice like a champion.

Play like a champion.

Live like a champion.

When exercising with JustHuynh fitness or performing our routines at home, in public, or at a gym, embrace the Commodore Creed so you can achieve at the highest level.

DOCTORS MINDSET FOR OBESITY ANTIDOTE

When I was skinny and weak, I couldn't defend myself or others. When I was fat, I was a drag to myself for not thriving in life and was a drag to society who had to pay for my healthcare costs, poor job performance, and low contribution to society.

The true measure of my life is how many lives I can positive change for the better. Evaluating fat loss options ranging from pills, to belly surgery, to fad diets, I realized that exercise is the natural antidote to become healthy. You too can make this happen if make exercise a habit just like brushing your teeth. With exercise as a habit, you will never again be a victim to the annual vicious cycle of getting fat where Americans tend to eat lots of food during Thanksgiving and Christmas, set New Year's fitness resolution in January, quit the gym in February, stay at home to watch TV in the cold Winter, go on vacation from April to August during the warm weather, and busy from September to November with back-to-school or end of year business.

JUSTHUYNH - BORN IN BOSTON - TITLETOWN

JustHuynh is pronounced "Just" + "Win" with our mission of helping people "Just Win" at health by training together. As an Asian American "model minority" who has overcome being discriminated against for being Asian, skinny, fat, dumb, shy, weak, and unfit, I've been able to channel a "huynhing/winning" mindset.

Some of the "just win" mentality has to do with being born in New England where we cheer on football's New England Patriots, basketball's Boston Celtics, and baseball's Boston Red Sox. With so many championships won, Boston has been labelled "City of Champions" and "Titletown USA" from being "Hungry to Huynh (Win)" despite their numerous titles. The reason fans "hate" Boston teams is because they're jealous of sustained championship greatness - wishing their hometown sports teams could steal that winning DNA. In baseball, it's New York (Yankees) vs Boston (Red Sox). In basketball, it's Los Angeles (Lakers) vs Boston (Celtics). And in football, it's New England (Patriots) vs the World (all the other NFL teams who want to be the Patriots). As you see, sports in North America revolves around Boston - a historical city in April 19, 1775 where the American Revolution began with the "Shot Heard Round the World."

In football, owner Bob Kraft, Coach Bill Belichick, and Quarterback Tom Brady have won 5 Super Bowls and played in 9 Super Bowl Games from 2001-2019 as the New England Patriots are always playing chess when the rest of the teams are playing checkers. Overlooked players like Julian Edelman gladly take less pay and play with a "f--k you" attitude, per Jerry Rice, for a chance to be called "Champion" with the greatest football player of all time Tom Brady - known for his "clutch" gene.

In basketball, the Boston Celtics own the most NBA Titles in NBA history with 17 NBA Championships. With only 5 people on the court at once, the Boston Celtics started a "Big 3" trend where three star players set aside their individual egos for the betterment of the team to "JustHuynh" championships. Bill Russell, Bob Cousy, and Tom Heinsohn won 6 NBA Championships together. Larry Bird, Kevin McHale, and Robert Parish won 3 NBA Championships together while facing Michael Jordan's Chicago Bulls, Isiah Thomas' Detroit Pistons, and Magic Johnson's Los Angeles Lakers. Paul Pierce, Kevin Garnett, and Ray Allen won 1 NBA Championship together that brought the Celtics back to relevance. The 2018 Big 3 was unique in that all 3 players were in their 30s, made multiple all-star teams, owned franchise scoring records, possessed a supportive fan base, and possessed 100 million dollar contracts. What was missing was a championship. All three hated being called "losers" as players are remembered for how many championships they win so all 3 realized it made sense to join forces in putting aside individual statistics for collective sacrifice of becoming a champion. The Boston Celtics' "Big 3" concept inspired the concept where players stuck in loser organizations form super teams to chase championships such as LeBron James did in Miami (Dwayne Wade and Chris Bosh) and Cleveland (Kyrie Irving and Kevin Love) while Kevin Durant joined the Golden State Warriors (Stephen Curry, Klay Thompson, and Draymond Green) who just had the best regular season record in NBA history with 73 wins to 9 losses.

In baseball, the Boston Red Sox killed the "Curse of the Bambino" which was a championship drought that lasted for 86 years since 1918. Since that curse-breaking World Series title in 2004, the Boston Red Sox have had the most championships with 4. Each of these 4 teams had players hungry to win championships. The 2018 World Series title was a great example of a "just win" mentality to take down big market teams in New York, Houston, and Los Angeles. After one victory by the New York Yankees in the Divisional Series, star Aaron Judge insulted the players in Boston by playing Frank Sinatra's "New York, New York" song by the Boston Red Sox locker room. Angered, the Boston Red Sox won the next two games to finish off the Yankees and move on to face the Houston Astros in the AL Championship Series (ALCS). Heading into Game 3 of the ALCS tied 1-1, star Alex Bregman teased Game 3 pitcher Nathan Eovaldi by posting an Instagram video showing Nathan Eovaldi giving up three straight home runs to Astros sluggers. Bregman immediately deleted the video when his teammates warned him to not anger the Red Sox, but the damage was already done with the Red Sox winning the remaining 3 games to make the World Series against the Los Angeles Dodgers. After losing Game 3 which was the longest game in postseason history at 18 innings over 7 hours and 20 minutes, the Boston Red Sox loss all energy after intended Game 4 pitcher Nathan Eovaldi was scratched from the start to pitch the most epic relief in history to save the Red Sox bullpen. So when Yasiel Puig flexed his muscles after hitting a 3 run home-run to potentially tie the World Series at 2-2, normally quiet star pitcher Chris Sale fired up his teammates by insulting his team's inability to kill an average opposing pitcher in Rich Hill screaming "Rich Hill has 2 f--king pitches." Motivated the Red Sox won game 4 and game 5 to become World Series Champions.

Like the "championship" and "winning" mindset of New England sports teams, JustHuynh Fitness' mission is to boost members' confidence and health so they can be champions and winners in life and business.

AGELESS SUPERCENTENARIAN PRINCIPLES

Have fun and laugh positively
Family is #1 - Enjoy life and love with a wife or husband
Avoid unhealthy habits of alcohol, drugs, smoking, fat foods, yo yo diets
Limit your time on TV, social media, video games
Pursue your passions to make the world a better place
Boost brain power thru reading or listening
Get at least 6 hours of sleep
Eat 1,500-1,800 calories daily with proper macronutrients

AGELESS JEFF BEZOS MOTIVATION SPEECH

There are many reasons that we want to live long healthily and happily such as being able to spend more time with our family and pursuing our passions. Jeff Bezos of Amazon is well-respected for being the fearless leader of 566,000 employees and delivering a superb Amazon Prime service to 100 million customers. In a YouTube Video titled "One of the Greatest Speeches Ever" Jeff Bezos delivers a motivational speech that should inspire you to live life purposefully saying "You guys will find out that you have passion. When you find that passion, it will be a gift for you because passion gives you purpose. You could have a job, you could have a career, or you could have a calling, and the best thing is to have a calling. If you find your passion, you'll have that calling where your work won't feel like work...You have to always be leaning into the future. If you lean away, the future is going to win everytime...Inventors have a paradoxical ability to have 10,000 hours of domain expertise and a beginner's mindset to look at situations with a fresh perspective....Don't chase what the hot passion of the day is because you'll end up unhappy. Instead, project yourself forward to Age 80 and envision looking back on your life to minimize the number of regrets. That works for career and family decisions. I have a 16 month old boy right now and would regret the rest of my life if wasn't there for my son's childhood."

Everyone has a calling, whether it's becoming the U.S. President like Barack Obama, a TV host like Ellen DeGeneres, a CEO like Jeff Bezos, a singer like Taylor Swift, a movie star like LeBron James, a sports star like Michael Jordan, a social media star like Kim Kardashian, a soldier, a teacher, a police, a doctor - just don't be a bully in life.

Looking to age 80, my calling is to boost people's confidence and self defense thru JustHuynh Fitness' martial arts and power athletics. I also aspire to raise accomplished children who can contribute to society even more than I will. What's your calling and vision?

ATHLETIC SUPERSTAR PRINCIPLES

Strength train 3 times a week for bone strength
Martial arts 3 times a week for heart health
Dominate the exercise room to thrive in bedroom and boardroom
Keep waist size under 40 inches for men and under 35 for women
Keep your BMI between 18.5 to 24.9
Remember obesity leads to diabetes, disease, depression, death
Dedicate time to warm-up and recover
Sprint 300 meters under 52.5 seconds (men) and 65 seconds (women)

ATHLETIC DREW BREES MOTIVATION SPEECH

In athletics, you are often training to be a "better you" in order to get personal records in a challenge or win a championship with a team. Football is one of the best team sports involving 53 players where the ability to lead a team can translate into leading a business with a similar amount of employees. In 2010, New Orleans Saints Quarterback Drew Brees was hailed as a hero for winning the city's first Super Bowl which had tremendous meaning as it was still suffering from Hurricane Katrina in 2005. Drew Brees came to the rescue again in delivering a "Lethal" pre-game speech during the 2019 NFL NFC Divisional Playoff game against the defending Super Bowl Champion Philadelphia Eagles that resulted in the Saints winning. Channel this energy every time you exercise or compete.

"Hey listen to me now. There's three stages to this game. You play, you compete, and you're lethal. When you're a kid, you play. You play because you love this game. Then you started learning fundamentals. You started learning technique. You started learning how to compete and how to win. Then the third stage - not everybody gets to the third stage. Not everybody gets to be lethal. But when you get a group of guys that love one another and plays for one another - that's lethal. When you go into every game and find a way to win no matter the circumstance - that's lethal. All season long we played, we competed, and tonight - we are lethal! Let's go baby. Win on three - 1,2,3 - WIN!"

ASSASSIN SUPERHERO PRINCIPLES

Avoid fights if can - if your life is in danger, fight or flight in under 90 seconds
Channel anger against trolls, traitors, and tools for superhuman performance
Adopt a formless fighting style when using your 8 limbs as a human weapon
Gain strength and respect the heartbreak that martial arts founders overcame
Prevent bullying and sexual assaults
Build a community to protect each other against hand, knife, and gun combat
Share martial arts with good souls regardless of their skin color

ASSASSIN BRUCE LEE MOTIVATION SPEECH

When faced with a life threatening situation, you must be able to eliminate the opponent to save your life. Bruce Lee is the only actor to have made the most impact in the world dead vs alive. As a Eurasian who was finally approved by Chinese masters to teach martial arts to non-Asians such as white martial artist Chuck Norris and black martial artist Jim Kelly, Bruce Lee inspired billions of short, weak, minority, and shy people that martial arts can help them thrive personally (Bruce Lee was loved by many Hollywood actresses) and professionally (many Hollywood actors wanted to learn martial arts and movie directors wanted to cast him in blockbuster films).

On the Pierre Berton Show and book titled "Tao of Jeet Kune Do," Bruce Lee, who has taught martials arts to actors James Gardner, Steve McQueen, Lee Marvin, Roman Polanski, and James Coburn says "I hope martial artists are more interested in the root of martial arts and not the different decorative branches, flowers, or leaves. It is futile to argue as to which single leaf, which design of branches or which attractive flower you like; when you understand the root, you understand all its blossoming...In fighting with no rules, you better train every part of your body."

CHARITABLE CAUSES JUSTHUYNH SUPPORTS

JustHuynh supports causes that help the world become Ageless Athletic Assassins. For ageless, JustHuynh supports anti-ageing and mental health. For athletics, JustHuynh supports reducing obesity and athletic development. For assassin, JustHuynh supports anti-bullying, rape prevention, and empowering Asian Americans to shatter the "Model Minority Bamboo Ceiling."

CHAPTER 7

MARTIAL ARTS FOR LIFE

A good plan violently executed now is better than a perfect plan executed next week

- General George S. Patton

FIT FOR YOUR JOB

Martial arts strengthens your body and mind. If you can focus on your conditioning, endurance, speed, power, balance, coordination, and agility, you'll be able to thrive personally, professionally, academically, and athletically. Martial arts is the best cardio and cross-training you need and JustHuynh Fitness' training program can help you unlock your potential like men and women in numerous professions have benefited from.

WOMEN #METOO & RAPE DEFENSE

Larger and stronger men often target women in sexual assaults such as rape assuming women can't defend themselves. Judo founder Kano Jigoro inspired United Kingdom women in 1910 who were physically beaten by police and men. By studying martial arts such as judo, woman who had average height of 4 ft 11 inches were able to defend themselves against men who had average height of 5 ft 10 inches. Female Shaolin Five Elder legend Ng Mui, who's Wing Chun fighting style has been passed down to Bruce Lee and Bruce's master Ip man, is most famous for teaching a 15-year old Chinese girl from being kidnapped.

In 2019, a women from Charlotte North Carolina, is forever grateful for martial arts when she ran into a karate dojo to escape a large 47-year-old black man from kidnapping her at 9PM. When the kidnapper tried to push by the karate master Randall Ephraim inside the studio in order to kidnap the women, the karate master used self defense saying "I then went into action defending myself and got him out of the dojo. Once outside he attempted to attack again and was dealt with accordingly." When the police arrived, the kidnapper was carried out of the dojo on a stretcher in pain. The woman and city lauded the karate master a "hero" for protecting the woman.

Women between the ages of 15 and 30 are most susceptible to date rape, muggings, kidnapping, and other assaults when they are out late at night especially if the night venue is located in unsafe areas. The Centers for Disease and Control and Prevention conducted a "National Intimate Partner and Sexual Violence Survey" in 2012 revealing that one in four women will be assaulted in their lifetime.

A study, conducted by the New England Journal of Medicine lead author Charlene Sene, compared the effects of attending a four session course totalling 12 hours in resisting sexual assault to a university approach of providing brochures on sexual assault. 451 freshman women from Canada universities took sessions including recognizing potential sexual assault scenarios and two hours of self defense training in martial arts. The 442 other women were the control group that received a 15 minute sexual assault session with a take-home brochure. One year after the self defense vs the brochure training, 9.8% of the brochure attendants had been raped whereas the sexual assault participants had lower rape percentage of 5.2%. Thus lead investigator Charlene says "Sexual assault prevention programs cuts risk of rape by nearly 50%. It's critical to give women the tools they need to fight back, however we also need to hold men accountable for sexual violence to cut down the number of sexual assault victims."

In 2019 a would be mugger tried to sexually assault 115 pound Polyana Viana but chose the wrong person as Polyana knows self defense martial arts as a UFC Fighter. Polyana said "I knew how to defend myself. He was really close to me. If it's a gun, he won't have time to draw it. I stood up. I threw two punches to his face and a kick. When he fell, I put him in a rear-naked choke. Then I sat him down to wait for the police."

It's very important to remember safety precautions such as not leaving a drink unattended or letting someone else get one for you, not walking alone, not walking distracted texting or talking on the phone, putting your car keys or sharp object between your fingers as a self-defense weapon, carrying an umbrella or belt as an extra self defense weapon, knowing where to kick and strike the attacker before running for safety.

For hand to hand self defense, the most efficient places to strike an attacker are the temple, eyes, jaw, nose, throat, neck, solar plexus, liver, ribs, groin, shins, knees, and feet. Practice these moves over and over again until your self defense reactions become natural: palm of the hand to the nose, hook punch or spinning hook kick to temple, finger to the eye, inside elbow to the jaw, punch to the throat, karate chop to neck, side kick to the solar plexus, left kick or left body punch to person's right rib cage, roundhouse or knee the ribs, front kick to the groin, roundhouse kick to the knees, side kick the shins, and heel stomp on the foot. Unarmed skills are the first and last line of defense. If you lose your weapon such as your gun, knife, or stick in a fight, unarmed hand combat skills are what keeps you alive. That's why the military forces train in unarmed close-quarters combat.

On the East Coast during the 1960s serial raper and killer named Albert DeSalvo known as the "Boston Strangler," who was a former soldier in the army, targeted random single women across Massachusetts from age 19 to age 85. The Boston Strangler's mode of operation was to gain entry into woman's home by saying he needed help for his broken car or that he was a detective before raping women and then killing them with the clothes they wore such as their belt and nylon stockings. Albert would leave all the raped and murdered victims on the floor fully naked with the strangulation item used placed around the woman's neck in a bow-tie shape. In 2013, the Boston Strangler's identity was finally solved after 50 years. The unsolved mystery inspired a 1968 Hollywood movie called "The Boston Strangler."

Over on the West Coast in California, a serial rapist and killer known as the "Golden State Killer and East Area Rapist" named Joseph DeAngelo, who was a police officer, terrorized Sacramento California from 1975 to 1986 - raping 50 women and killing 13 women. Joseph targeted married women living in middle-class neighborhoods at night. Joseph performed research of the victims beforehand by peeping thru windows before entering homes unnoticed to unlock windows, unload guns, plant weapons for his later use, and call women to understand their daily routines. Finally in 2018, investigators used DNA evidence to arrest Joseph DeAngelo. Authorities said "The serial killer would monitor suburban neighborhoods and sneak into homes at night. If a couple was home, he would tie up the man, place dishes on his back and threaten to kill both victims if he heard the plates fall onto the floor while he raped the woman repeatedly for several hours." Writer Michelle McNamara wrote a book about the search for the Golden State Killer called "I'll Be Gone In The Dark" which will be produced into an HBO docuseries.

In 2015 in Melbourne Australia, 25-year old Taela Davis was enjoying an afternoon walk with her earphones in until she was attacked from behind and thrown on the ground by a 6 foot tall man with the intent to rape her. Fortunately, Taela's black belt in karate helped her defend herself as she punched him in the face until he bled, kneed him in the ribs, and headbutted him - finally escaping when a male passerby came over that caused the bloody man to run away. Her Karate Master Ennio Ans was proud that his students used their training to escape a dangerous situation saying "When I test students for their black belts we have a survival test that involves the student being unexpectedly attacked by another club member with a black belt. They have 90 seconds to break free and get away. This training is what Taela used to escape a real-life attack." Tracee Hall-Davis, Taela's mom, is proud that she made both daughters take karate saying "I'd recommend martial arts for all women. It's good to have the skills to defend yourself."

MEN ANTI-BULLYING DEFENSE

In Japan during the late 1800s weak men such as Karate founder Gichin Funakoshi couldn't learn martial arts because the government enforced laws forbidding the teaching of martial arts as the government viewed "hands and feet" as weapons that could be used to challenge the government. United States General Douglas MacArthur also banned Japanese martial art forms Judo and Kendo in 1945 after the end of World War II because the United States viewed martial artists as a violent threat. Fortunately, Karate was permitted to be taught as the discipline was classified as "physical education not martial arts" - allowing Karate to spread in the United States during the 1950s when American soldiers opened karate dojos.

In the face of war, men used martial arts to defend their country such as in Thailand especially during the 1760s when the "Father of Muay Thai" Nai Khanom impressed enemy Burmese Lord Mangra by defeating 10 consecutive elite Burmese fighters. In South Korea, civilians were banned from being taught martial arts similar to what was experienced in Japan, until the government lifted the martial arts ban after World War II. Civilians loved Taekwondo for its heavy emphasis on using the legs that gave people a reach advantage over people who only knew how to use their hands.

Israel was inspired by Japanese judo and aikido which saved lives in the 1930s when anti-Semitic groups attacked the Jewish community. That's when the "Father of Krav Maga" Imi Lichtenfeld taught Krav Maga to a group of men to defend their Jewish community against anti-Semitic thugs.

Men would fare well in life-threatening hand-to-hand combat if they were able to execute martial arts moves from notable movie scenes such as the "Mission: Impossible -- Fallout" Bathroom Fight Scene where Asian Kung Fu martial artist Liang Yang takes on Krav Maga practitioner Tom Cruise and Brazilian Jiu Jitsu practitioner Henry Cavill, "IP Man" IP man vs Japanese General fight scene that features Donnie Yen's Wing Chun against karate, "Way of the Dragon" Bruce Lee's Jeet Kune Do vs Chuck Norris' karate, "The Raid Redemption" featuring Mad Dog vs Rama and Andi, and "Fist of Legend" Jet Li vs General fight scene.

However since the Sandy Hook Elementary School mass shooting in Connecticut killed 26 people in 2012, there have been 1,929 mass shootings from then until the end of year 2018. You could be susceptible to the presence of an active shooter anywhere you go such as we saw at a gay Orlando nightclub in 2016 where a 29-year old security guard killed 49 people and wounded 53 others, at an outdoor concert in Las Vegas in 2017 where a real estate investor fired more than 1,100 rounds of ammunition from the 32nd floor of the Mandalay Bay hotel that killed 58 people and injured 851 people, at a movie theatre in Colorado in 2012 where a mentally ill shooter killed 12 and injured 58 people, at a synagogue in Pittsburgh in 2018 where an anti-semitic shooter killed 11 and injured 7 people of the Jewish community, at a mall in Nebraska in 2007 where a mentally-ill shooter killed 8 people, at a McDonald's in San Diego in 1984 where a mentally ill man killed 21 and injured 19 people, at a nursing home in North Carolina in 2009 where a depressed shooter killed a nurse and 7 elderly people, at a workplace office in San Francisco in 1993 where a depressed shooter killed 9 and injured 6 people, at a company holiday party with 80 people in 2015 in San Bernardino where a violent couple killed 14 and injured 24 people, at a college campus at Virginia Tech in 2007 where a mentally-ill student used two semi-automatic pistols to kill 31 and injure 17 people, and at a high school in Florida where a mentally ill shooter killed 17 adults and children.

In Nashville Tennessee in 2018 at 3:25AM, caught inside the bloodbath at a Waffle House where an active shooter had already killed 4 people and injured 4 more, 29-year-old James Shaw Jr heroically stayed alive and saved dozens of other's lives by running forward to slam a swivel door at the active shooter while he was reloading his AR-15 assault rifle. This caused the shooter to run away. James was mentally prepared to take advantage of this situation as 11 children were able to escape the 2012 Sandy Hook Elementary school mass shooting when the active shooter paused to reload per Nicole Hockley whose six-year old son was killed at Sandy Hook. Whenever you sense that a mentally-ill shooter is reloading, that is your opportunity to save your life by escaping or attempting a physical tackle. Many described James as a hero but he didn't agree saying "I was completely doing it just to save myself. After the shooter shot thru the swivel door, I knew there was no way to lock the swivel door so made up my mind that if it was going to come down to it that the shooter was going to have to work to kill me."

Taking action to save his life is a must with no guarantee that police would arrive in time. Waffle House CEO said "I personally want to thank Mr. Shaw. You don't get to meet too many heroes in life. You're my hero. You saved people's lives and they will thank you for the rest of their lives." He even inspired "Black Panther" actor Chadwick Boseman to hand his MTV "Best Superhero" award to James saying that James is the "real life" hero.

Most of the mass shootings were conducted by men with mental health issues that wanted to kill as many people as possible before committing suicide. Some shooters targeted particular demographics such as people from the Jewish (Pittsburgh Synagogue) and gay (Orlando nightclub) communities. In an age where celebrities with millions of followers on Instagram or Twitter can influence followers, everyone must be sure that commonly targeted groups aren't hurt. For instance in 2018 comedian Kevin Hart, who has 35 million Twitter and 68 million Instagram followers, made a series of homophobic posts such as "If my son comes home & plays with my daughter's doll house, I'm going to break it over his head & say 'stop that's gay'." This angered the gay community causing Kevin Hart to step down from hosting the 2018 Oscars and gay celebrities such as CNN news anchor Don Lemon asked for Kevin to apologize and help the gay community feel welcome. In 2018 LeBron James, who has 46 million Instagram followers, upset the Jewish community with his Instagram Story post saying "We been getting that Jewish money, Everything is Kosher." This is personal to the Jewish community who have been targeted by the Nazis since the Holocaust resulting in the death of six million Jews. "Entourage" producer Doug Ellin took offense with LeBron saying "This is an anti-Semitic stereotype used for centuries to foster hatred against Jews. @kingjames the Nazis spread this nonsense everywhere #wordshavemeaning posting words to 44 million people has a ton of meaning." This anti-semitic post was shortly after an earlier post LeBron James made about NBA and NFL owners saying "In the NFL they got a bunch of old white men owning teams and they got that slave mentality. And it's like, 'This is my team. You do what the f**k I tell y'all to do. Or we get rid of y'all'." The lesson here is whether you have 0 followers or millions of followers like Kevin Hart and LeBron James to treat all humans with respect or else you condone hate speech against targeted demographics.

POLITICIAN ANTI-VIOLENCE DEFENSE

World leaders understand the importance of being physically fit. Taking the cue from Russian President Vladimir Putin who practices Judo,

President Barack Obama trained in Taekwondo in Chicago, IL when he was a part-time state senator and was awarded an honorary black belt by South Korean president Lee Myung-Bak in 2009.

To treat asthma, President Theodore Roosevelt practiced Judo and President George H.W. Bush practiced Taekwondo with "the Father of American Taekwondo" Jhoon Rhee. Jhoon Rhee was legendary as he was inspired to train United States politicians as Americans helped the South Koreans when the North Koreans attempted to invade South Korea after World War II. Jhoon realized politicians needed martial arts training when Rep. James Cleveland (R-NH) was mugged one night so Jhoon phoned Rep Cleveland letting him know that he'd never get mugged again if he learned martial arts. This was the birth of the Congressional Tae Kwon Do Club who trained Mondays, Wednesdays, and Fridays at 6:30AM. Over a 45 year span, Jhoon Rhee trained 350 politicians including Reps. Gene Taylor (D-MS), Gregory Meeks (D-NY), John Adler (D-NJ), Earl Pomeroy (D-ND), Mike McIntyre (D-NC), Pete Hoekstra (R-MI), Carolyn Maloney (D-NY), Jesse Jackson, Jr. (D-IL), Vice President Biden when he served in the Senate, House Speakers Newt Gingrich (R-GA), Tom Foley (D-WA), Sen. Ted Stevens (R-AK), Rep. Silvio Conte (R-MA), Sen Milton Young (R-ND), and Sen Joseph Montoya (D-NM).

CEO BLACK BELTS

CEOs understand the benefits martial arts provides physically and mentally for business.

Nasdaq CEO Adena Friedman is a leading Wall Street figure who was inspired to take Taekwondo after watching her children take martial arts classes. Instead of just sitting on the sidelines watching her children, Adena made Taekwondo a family activity in achieving her black belt saying "My lessons from Taekwondo is to use your strength to do the right thing. Lots of lessons that you can apply to business."

Intuit CEO Brad Smith credits much of his success to the discipline he gained through his martial arts training in karate as a young man. Brad says "I learned at an early age through my martial arts training—where, as a black belt and teacher, you are measured on the progress of your students—that I loved getting things done through a team as opposed to going solo."

PayPal CEO Dan Schulman attributes his career success to practicing krav maga everyday saying "I think what I really love about martial arts is there's a lot of philosophy around it. The biggest thing that you're taught is there are all sorts of ways of de-escalating fighting situations...confidence also carries over to business."

Palantir CEO Alex Karp credits practicing qigong in helping him build the 'Killer App' that helped catch terrorist Osama bin Laden. As a 51 year old billionaire bachelor, Alex is so focused on using data, technology, and human expertise to help law enforcement and intelligence agencies causing him to say "The only time I'm not thinking about Palantir is when I'm swimming, practising Qigong or having sex."

Although Silicon Valley CEOs Mark Zuckerberg of Facebook, Sundar Pichai of Google, and Jeff Weiner of Linkedin are not martial artists, all provide their employees martial arts courses for self defense with Facebook & Google offering brazilian jiu jitsu and Linkedin offering muay thai classes. All companies say martial arts empowers staff with knowledge of self defense, healthy living, stress relief, and team productivity.

HOLLYWOOD ACTION STARS

As a movie star, an amazing body helps actors and actresses stand out on the big screen. Martial arts is the best way to help actors and actresses get an amazing physique and fighting skills.

In "Wonder Woman," Gal Gadot trained six hours a day - 2 hours martial arts, 2 hours horseback riding, and 2 hours of fighting sequences. In "Suicide Squad," Margot Robbie practiced brazilian jiu jitsu 3 times a week, boxing 4 times a week, and gymnastics 3.5 times a week. In "Million Dollar baby," Hilary Swank credits krav maga in providing her the best physique and fighting form. For a personal challenge, Idris Elba trained 12 months in Muay Thai for his first professional fight. For the "Matrix" and "John Wick," Keanu Reeves practice brazilian jiu-jitsu, judo, knife fighting, and tactical gun work. In "Kill Bill," Uma Thurman and her co-stars trained in Kung Fu 8 hours a day Monday thru Friday for 3 months straight. For "Mission Impossible" and "Jack Reacher," Tom Cruise practiced krav maga to quickly take down attackers with knives and guns. In "The Debt," Jessica Chastain practiced krav maga 2 hours a day for 4 months straight. "Sherlock Holmes" star Robert Downey Jr. and "Batman" star Christian Bale both practiced Wing Chun 6 days a week. In "Buffy the Vampire Slayer," Sarah Michelle Gellar trained in Taekwondo, kickboxing, boxing and street-fighting. In "Only God Forgives," Ryan Gosling trained Muay Thai two hours a day for four days a week. Power couple Brad Pitt and Angelina Jolie both practiced krav maga 45 minutes a day to gain muscle, lose fat, and improve overall health.

Physical bullying is one of the most disgraceful actions someone can do especially if you're a martial artist. When you bully someone, that person is destroyed physically and mentally where suicidal thoughts or depression might arise. In 2019 actor Jonah Hill made an Instagram post about being bullied in high school and how martial arts has improved his life and health saying "I started Brazilian Jiu Jitsu 2 months ago and train 4 or 5 times a week. In high school the dudes who did Jiu Jitsu used to beat the s**t out of us...At 35, I get over stuff that made me feel weak and insecure as a teenager." Kudos to Jonah for overcoming his fears thru martial arts.

Most powerful is how martial arts can change your life in eliminating bad habits such as alcohol, poor nutrition, smoking, and drug addiction. Former Sopranos star Michael Imperioli credits martial arts for changing his life, his wife Victoria, and his children. Michael says "I was in terrible physical shape. I smoked a pack a day...I have more focus, concentration, and confidence...Taekwondo teaches you that you can overcome any obstacle."

BILLBOARD SINGER MARTIAL ARTISTS

In the music industry, The Mind Freak practices kung-fu, karate, and taekwondo; Rolling Stones Mick Jagger trains judo, Elvis Presley had a black belt in karate, Kylie Minogue practice Taekwondo, Michael Jackson did kung fu, Jennifer Lopez trained in krav maga for "Enough" film, the Wu Tang Clan was inspired by Bruce Lee to take Kung Fu, Madonna did karate with her then-husband Guy Ritchie, Usher practices Muay Thai, Demi Lovato does brazilian jiu jitsu, and Wiz Khalifa does Muay Thai.

TV HOSTS FIT FOR SHOW TIME

Stars in TV Show Business realize that martial arts can help them look great on television. CNN's 48 year old host Chris Cuomo wakes up at 3:30 a.m. to do mixed martial arts and lifting. Chris focuses on practical self-defense moves so he's ready for scenarios when attacked. He loves the ability to defend himself and his family.

Podcast host Joe Rogan trains Taekwondo, Brazilian jiu-jitsu, and Muay Thai which prepared him when former martial artist Wesley Snipes challenged Joe Rogan to an MMA fight, but backed out after discovering Joe Rogan knows Taekwondo.

"Price is Right" host Bob Barker is a karate black belt who learned his sidekicks from Chuck Norris.

COMEDIAN MARTIAL ARTISTS

Comedians with martial arts can defend themselves against critics. Kevin Hart practices hand combat in his Instagram posts.

As a tall 300 pound man, Dante Nero practices Jeet Kune Do, Brazilian Jiu Jitsu, Karate, and Krav Maga.

Comedian W. Kamau Bell, inspired by Bruce Lee's philosophy, does kung fu and taekwondo. In the "Fist of Fury," Kamau admires Bruce Lee for challenging and defeating Japanese fighters to proclaim the worth of Chinese people during the Sino-Japanese wars.

VICTORIA'S SECRET FIGHT BODY

Victoria's Secret models know that martial arts help you tone and lose fat fast. Tom Brady's wife Gisele Bundchen practices kung fu and tai chi, legendary Adriana Lima does boxing and kickboxing, Lilian Dikmans practices Muay Thai in Australia, and Devon Windsor does kickboxing.

NFL FOOTBALL DOOMSDAY DEFENSE

Martial arts helps football players stay in shape while improving their hand positioning and foot agility in games. NFL Pass Rushers benefit as hand combat is the art of creating leverage with strategic hand placement at the line of scrimmage - allowing pass rushers to terrorize quarterbacks after they outsmart the bigger offensive linemen. The New England Patriots, Cleveland Browns, Kansas City Chiefs, Washington Redskins and Chicago Bears have employed martial arts specialists to give them an edge against the competition.

Before coming to the New England Patriots, Bill Belichick was the New York Giants defensive coordinator from 1985 to 1990 where he noticed pass rushers Lawrence Taylor and Andre Tippett destroying everyone on the field. After learning Lawrence and Andre both used their martial arts training in games, Bill Belichick hired Joe Kim as an assistant strength coach when he took the Cleveland Browns head coaching job. Knowing Joe Kim was a fourth-degree black belt and a member of the United States National Taekwondo team, Bill assigned Joe Kim to work with the team's pass rushers that helped defensive end Anthony Pleasant go from 4 sacks in 1992 to 11 in 1993. As the head coach of the New England Patriots since 2000, Bill Belichick has used martial arts to achieve 5 Super Bowl Championships.

In 1977, before Joe Kim, Bruce Lee's famous training partner and student Dan Inosanto was brought on by Cowboy's conditioning coach Bob Ward to run a secret martial arts training program for the Dallas Cowboys. Inosanto's martial arts training led to the Dallas Cowboys Super Bowl Champion "Doomsday Defense." A film on the Cowboys Defense produced by Inosanto's daughter Diana says "I always thought people should know my dad's responsibility for being the first man to introduce martial arts into the NFL and how it was secretly used. This was an East-meets-West experiment that had electrifying results that would carry down the line in football."

Other NFL players benefiting from martial arts are D'Brickashaw Ferguson who is a black belt in karate with improved coordination and discipline, Jared Allen who got a career high 15.5 sacks in 2007 by training mixed martial arts, Clay Matthews practices mixed martial arts to condition his body and mind, DeMarcus Ware trains Muay Thai for quickness that helped him achieve 134.5 career sacks; Carlos Dunlap, Connor Barwin and Luke Kuechly all practice Kung Fu, boxing, judo, and jiu jitsu; Anthony Zettel started mixed martial arts in college at Penn State University, Datone Jones says MMA training helps his hand-eye coordination, balance, body control, hand striking, endurance, and flexibility; Vikings Brian Robison says MMA techniques helps him rush the quarterback, and even San Francisco 49ers kicker David Akers practices jiu-jitsu, Shaolin Kempo, and Karate.

BASEBALL AIKIDO HOME-RUN KINGS

Martial arts helps baseball players with hand-eye coordination and agility on the field.

Sadaharu Oh, who has 868 career home runs, struggled early in his career with the Yomiuri Giants until he met hitting coach Hiroshi Arakawa who fused the sword-based martial art of Aikido with baseball. Oh overcame the stereotype that "short and weak" Asians can't hit home runs.

Noting Sadaharu Oh's success, Cleveland Indians Francisco Lindor goes to Japan during the offseason to practice Aikido.

Cleveland Indians catcher Yan Gomes does martial arts three or four times each week in the morning. Yan becomes the "Yanimal" - warming up with shadow boxing, stances, footwork, and mitt work to improve reaction.

Adam Dunn does boxing and kickboxing to improve throwing, swinging, fitness, and mental strength.

Catcher Russell Martin does mixed martial arts six days a week to boost his endurance, increase explosiveness, and lose body fat.

Pitcher Brad Penny says MMA prepares him in the event a hitter rushes the mound.

Pitcher Ryan Rowland-Smith says MMA has helped him get in the shape of his life and increased his focus to strike out opposing hitters.

BASKETBALL BRUCE LEE MAMBA MENTALITY

Martial arts helps basketball players with the mentality to dominate against one-on-one matchups.

The most famous basketball player to benefit from martial arts is Los Angeles Lakers Kareem Abdul Jabbar who studied Jeet Kune Do under Bruce Lee and even starred in Bruce Lee's final film "Game of Death." Kareem credits martial arts in providing him the discipline needed to win six championships with the Los Angeles Lakers.

Young Los Angeles Lakers Kobe Bryant took notice and also practiced Jeet Kune Do - crediting Bruce Lee for his "Mamba Mentality" of winning five NBA championships with the Lakers.

Los Angeles Lakers great Shaquille O'Neal also benefited from martial arts - practicing boxing, Jiu-Jitsu, and Muay Thai that helped him win four NBA championships with the Los Angeles Lakers and the Miami Heat.

Carmelo Anthony hopes his martial arts will help him win an elusive first NBA championship saying "As athletes, and as basketball players, you have to find different things that can help you on the basketball court. For me, that's boxing. When I'm in the gym, it's me versus you and I don't want to leave that gym with a loss. So that goes into my mindset, and it puts me in that tenacious focus on the basketball court that you just don't want to lose."

Miami Heat James Johnson has the nickname "Blood Sport" as both his parents and 8 siblings are all karate black belts. When James played for the Chicago Bulls, Derrick Rose chose James Johnson as his roommate knowing his qualifications as a bodyguard and enforcer. Chris Paul challenged James saying "I keep hearing about your fighting, but you're way too big to be a fighter" so James did a roundhouse kick within inches of Chris' face causing Chris to step back and say "O.K. I believe you James." In 2018 against the Philadelphia 76ers, Ben Simmons and James Johnson tussled so Ben's teammates immediately pulled Ben aside knowing James' martial arts background. Twitter laughed at Ben's stupidity in challenging a karate black belt saying "In the span of an NBA quarter, James Johnson somehow managed to expose the entire Sixers team as fake tough guys - Incredible."

NHL HOCKEY FIGHT READY PLAYERS

Martial arts helps hockey players stay physically strong on the ice against aggressive opponents and possess a fighting foundation when they engage in a fight on the ice. Hockey players also improve their hands, breathing and balance.

Hundreds of NHL hockey players practice martial arts including New York Islanders Matt Martin, Dallas's Tyler Seguin, Philadelphia's Wayne Simmonds, Anaheim's Adam Henrique and Andrew Cogliano, St. Louis's Robby Fabbri, Buffalo's Jeff Skinner, Edmonton's Darnell Nurse; Pittsburgh's Sidney Crosby, Jamie Oleksiak, Ryan Strome, and Dylan Strome; Montreal's Max Domi.

Buffalo Sabres goalie Robin Lehner says "Mixed martial arts skills mimic read-and-reach elements needed in NHL, provide a more-engaging full-body workout, and readiness for the threat of an opponent looking to land punches and kicks in a brawl fight."

Boston Bruins 7 foot hockey player Zdeno Chara, the tallest NHL hockey player ever, is known around the NHL as a workout fanatic. Zdeno's agent Matt Keator says "He like his meats lean (ideally, eating rabbit), potato baked (no salt, butter, or sour cream), and veggies steamed (no dressing). Alcohol can lead to dehydration and decreased levels of testosterone so Zdeno stays away from alcohol. He also does wrestling and the martial art of aikido - dubbed as the most feared fighter in the NHL."

SOCCER STRIKER KICKBOXING STARS

Martial arts helps soccer players with scoring, footwork, agility, speed, and endurance. Swedish soccer superstar Zlatan Ibrahimovic earned a black belt in Taekwondo as a 17-year-old that has helped him score some of the most amazing goals ever such as his overhead bicycle kick from 30 yards against England in a 2012 friendly.

French superstar Paul Pogba is a lethal kickboxer who credits martial arts with helping him win France the 2018 World Cup and improving his soccer play with Manchester United.

English soccer star Wayne Rooney credits martial arts with his striking ability to become the youngest player at age 17 to represent England in international play - becoming England's all-time record goalscorer with 53 goals in 120 international caps.

GOLF MARTIAL ARTISTS

Martial arts helps golfers with swing power, hip turn for long drives, mental strength for put shots, and endurance to last the entire game. Motivated from critics calling him "out of shape," Phil Mickelson practiced kung fu and Taekwondo.

TENNIS MARTIAL ARTISTS

Martial arts helps tennis players with power shots, agility to catch drop shots, endurance for long matches, and ability to grunt strong.

Notable tennis players who practice martial arts are Andy Murray, Caroline Wozniacki, Victoria Azarenka, and Jim Kelly.

COLLEGE #METOO RAPE SELF DEFENSE

In America, college is a 4 year experience where students live outside of their homes for the first time in their lives. What parents and students should worry about is the chance of rape or bullying on campus especially when offenders are under the influence of alcohol. According to the 2014 federal campus safety data, 100 universities reported at least 10 rape incidents during the year with Brown University and the University Connecticut tied for the highest annual incidents at 43 rapes each. American Association of University Women VP for Government Relations Lisa Maatz says "Universities need to stop trying to treat rape as a PR problem and treat it as the civil rights and public safety issue that it is."

Jessica Valenti, author of "Sex Object: A Memoir" who's a graduate of Tulane University, cites a 2015 national poll conducted by the Kaiser Family Foundation that found men in fraternities are three times more likely to rape women and women in sororities are 74% more likely to experience rape than non-sorority women. Jessica cites examples of rape cultures across America to forewarn current and incoming college students such as at Yale University where fraternity brothers marched through campus yelling "No means yes, yes means anal," at Georgia Tech where a fraternity brother sent an email guide called "Luring your rapebait," and at Wesleyan University where a fraternity was nicknamed the "Rape Factory."

Being raped can ruin one's life forever even leading to suicide such as the tragic incidents at Rhodes University in 2018 when Khensani Maseko committed suicide after being raped by another student, at Dartmouth Canada in 2013 when Rehtaeh Parsons hung herself after she was gang raped by 4 males, at the University of Missouri in 2010 when Sasha Menu Courey committed suicide after being raped by three football players, at William Paterson University in 2016 when Cherelle Locklear committed suicide after being raped at a frat party, and at the University of Alabama Tuscaloosa in 2016 when Megan Rondini committed suicide after being raped by someone she met at a bar.

University of Windsor Professor Charlene Sene did a $1.3 million research test comparing results of women 1 year after 400 women college freshman took martial arts training vs 400 women college freshman who had a quick 15 minute session about sexual assault with results showing that sexual assault prevention programs reduce risk of rape by nearly 50%.

In the midst of the #MeToo Era, colleges and universities across the United States are required to detail how they deal with sexual assault as mandated by the U.S. Department of Education's 2013 Campus Sexual Violence Elimination Act or risk losing federal funding. From 1999-2013, the U.S. federal government spent over $139 million on over 388 projects to reduce sexual violence in their Campus Grant Program, but rape has not decreased. University of Windsor professor Charlene Senn developed a program called "Flip the Script" that has students recognize the most common sexual misconduct signals and defend themselves with martial arts. Students participating in the program have seen rapes reduced by 50% and attempted rapes by 63% 1 year after enrolling in the 12 hour class.

2014 Miss USA Nia Sanchez, who is a fourth-degree black belt in Taekwondo, amazes people with her martial arts. During the Miss USA competition, Nia used her platform to stress the importance for college-aged women to learn martial arts due to the high rate of sexual assault on campus. For self defense Nia says "Break their knee, break their ankle, break their elbow. Make sure they're in so much pain, they can't cause you any pain."

SCHOOL ANTI-VIOLENCE

Kindergarten thru 12th grade are important years of a child's life but bullying gets in the way of a safe school environment. A 2009 Zaidi study published in the Archives of General Psychiatry following 5,000 children in Finland found that boys and girls who get bullied were more likely than their peers to require psychiatric treatment in their teens or early 20s.

Hong Kong schools take anti-bullying seriously where children as young as age seven learn self defense. Eight-year-old Tallie Lin from a Hong

Kong School says "You have to learn to protect yourself in case you are kidnapped or someone tries to kill you with punches, kicks, chokes, knives, guns, or a kidnap attempt."

School shootings are a major problem in the United States. The most tragic incidents were in 2012 when a gunman killed 20 children, six adults, and himself at Sandy Hook Elementary School in Connecticut; and in 2018 when a gunman killed 17 people at Marjory Stoneman Douglas (MSD) High School in Parkland, Florida. Per gun control advocacy organization "Everytown For Gun Safety," there have been 300 school shootings in the United States from 2013 - 2019 or about 1 school shooting per week.

Many States and local municipalities have passed law allowing teachers to arm themselves. The best case scenario is for a school resource officer to take down an active shooter such as Dixon Public Schools police Officer Mark Dallas did in 2018 when he was honored as the "International Association of Chiefs of Police" Officer of the Year by President Donald Trump for saving his son and 182 classmates from an active shooter. However not all school resource officers fulfill their duty of protecting their school community's lives such as MSD Officer Scot Peterson who stayed outside instead of going inside the school to kill the gunman. In an interview with "Today" after Officer Peterson was forced to retire, Peterson said "I'm sorry." When resource officers fail to protect lives of the school community or resource officers get killed in action, the standard "Code Red" protocol for schools is to hide in a locked classroom with the lights turn off until police arrive. This strategy of "hiding" while waiting for police makes school's vulnerable to being killed by shooters since no one is in self defense mode to take down the attacker as a group.

Theodore Roosevelt once said, "In any moment of decision…the best thing you can do is the right thing, the next best thing is the wrong thing, and the worst thing you can do is nothing." The right thing to do in order to stay alive, is to use self defense with armed teachers or self defense via group attack or else everyone risks being killed before the police even come. Skeptical of a resource officer's commitment to protecting students, the Clarkesville School District in Arkansas told their community "arming teachers is more cost-effective to improving school safety than hiring a school resource officer. Instead of spending $50,000 a year on one school resource officer, we can train 13 school teachers to use a gun for $68,000 total."

According to a 2006 study from the American Academy of Pediatrics, 43% of school superintendents don't have a prevention plan for mass-shooting events and 33% have never conducted a mass shooting drill.

Many schools in the United States that do have mass shooting drills have training methods for high school age and below-high school age. For below-high school where students are generally younger than 15 years old, young kids can practice spreading out to throw classroom objects such as heavy textbooks at the shooter to knock them out. High school age children can tackle the shooter with their collective force.

ARMY SURVIVAL OF THE FITTEST

Survival on the battlefield is of utmost importance to staying alive. In 2018 when the United States Military realized that too many soldiers were unfit that lead to injuries and deaths in war, the U.S. Military created a new Army Fitness Combat Readiness Test to ensure all current and future soldiers have adequate strength and endurance to survive on the battlefield. China also realized the importance of fitness saying the country has experienced unprecedented levels of obesity with over 300 million obese Chinese.

The United States Military's interest in martial arts was high during the occupation of several East Asian nations after World War II when Americans were exposed to martial arts forms of Taekwondo and Karate. In South Korea, Americans learned valuable hand to hand fighting techniques for situations when soldiers did not have guns or were fighting in close quarters. In the 1960s during the Vietnam War against the North Vietnamese, American soldiers were awed and intimidated when they saw South Korean Marines kneed the opponent's ribs, snapped necks, choked the enemy to death, and used bone crushing elbow strikes. The North Vietnamese avoided combat with the elite South Korean marines due to the high kill-ratio.

POLICE CITY PROTECTORS

Police officers succeed when they can safely protect people who live in their city while using the appropriate amount of force needed to stop crime.

Japanese police force showed the United States Army the importance of martial arts knowledge when the Sagamihara South Police Station provided a demonstration (judo, kendo, karate) in 2012 to U.S. Army Japanese Soldiers and Japanese city officials. Sagamihara officers and officers from all cities in Japan perform demonstrations (Budo Hajime Shiki) annually to the public as a way to show the police's commitment to protecting their respective communities. Sagamihara South Police Deputy chief Masaichi Yuguchi says "martial arts training helps us overcome fear and gain confidence in the event when we must engage physically with a suspect. This demonstration is an opportunity to show our community that we are here to protect them and that our motivation to do so is very high."

Influenced by Bruce Lee's nunchaku usage in "Enter the Dragon" movie, Anderson California police department adopted the use of nunchucks for police officers to subdue suspects with less force than other police weapons such as the gun, baton, and stun guns. Chief Michael Johnson says "Nunchucks help as a grappling tool for pain compliance around a suspect's wrist, elbows, and ankles." Many applauded the Anderson California police department including comedian Stephen Colbert in his "Fear Not, Karate Cops Are Here" video where he warns officers "not to hurt themselves when they use nunchucks for attack as it takes more than 16 hours to be Bruce Lee level."

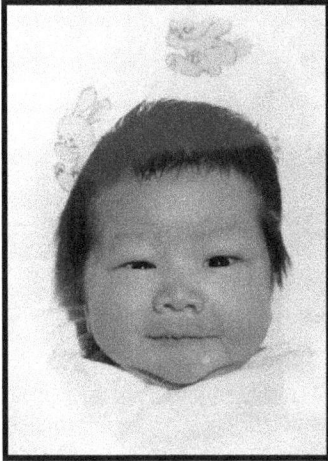

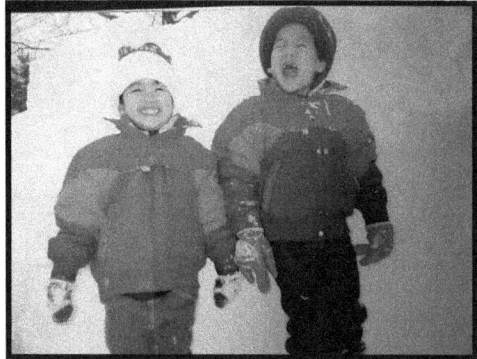

Above: Born August 23, 1988 (Year of the Dragon) in Portland, Maine. Named after Francis of Assisi by Father Gilbert, who sponsored my parents from Vietnam War, as a reminder to never forget about the poor due to my parents risking their lives as boat people coming to America with nothing. My dad named me Khang that means "strong."

Above: My brother Brian and I. Raised by parents who worked blue-collar low wage jobs who saved all their earnings so we could achieve the American Dream thru education

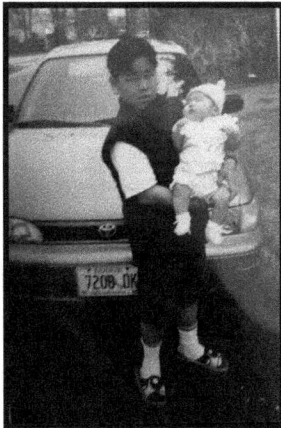

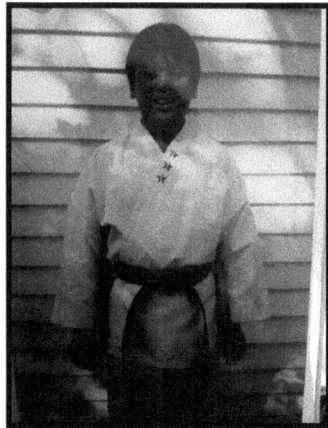

Above: Childhood obesity at age 10. Discriminated against and bullied in school for being fat, Asian, weak, slow, shy, and dumb.

Above: My father noticed poor grades in school and low self-esteem. Enrolling in martial arts improved my grades to graduate top 10 in high school and gain admission into #4 rank Bowdoin College

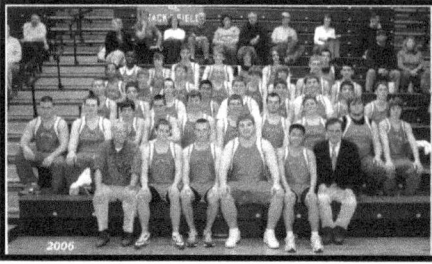

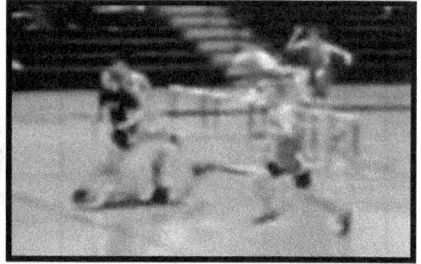

Above: socially shamed from youth sports due to being short 5ft2in, Asian, weak, fat, and unathletic, track is the only sport that doesn't cut athletes. Legendary South Portland High School coaches Paul Brogan and John Chapin transformed me thru sprinting and athletics

Above: youth athletes can sometimes feel invincible. This changed senior year of high school when I didn't stretch due to overconfidence of winning so I tripped over hurdle, blacked out for 10 minutes, pulled my hamstring, and lost an eyebrow

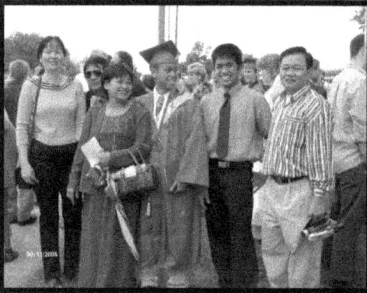

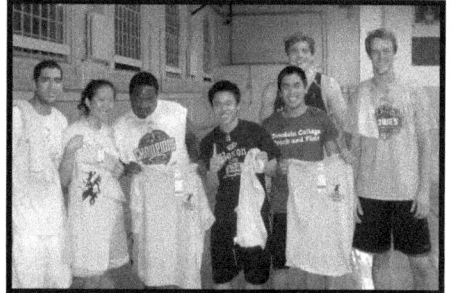

Above: achieved my parents high school goal for us: top 10 grades, Ivy-league caliber college (Bowdoin), leadership (captains for indoor and outdoor track), and community service (tutor young) - making their sacrifices worth it

Above: led the most diverse Bowdoin College club basketball team to a championship with 2 tall white centers, 2 black scorers, and 3 fast Asian defenders. Our team's name was "Just Put It In."

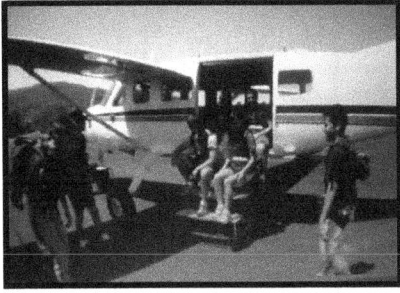

Above: during study abroad spring semester of junior year in college. Tested my bravery skydiving at 14,000 feet over the Great Barrier Reef in Australia. 1 person died the day before so we all said our prayers during the 3 hour van drive to the skydiving site. I was first to jump off the plane. One lady before us got a free skydive for falling naked

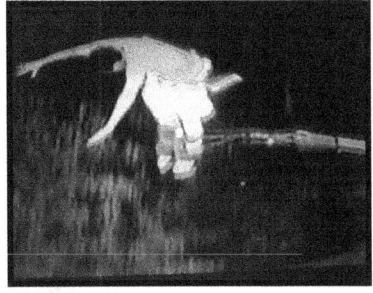

Above: the day after the skydive, did an AJ Hackett bungy jump with just a towel wrapped around my foot from a 50 meter tower. The same lady from the skydive got a free bungy jump for jumping naked while riding a bike off a roof

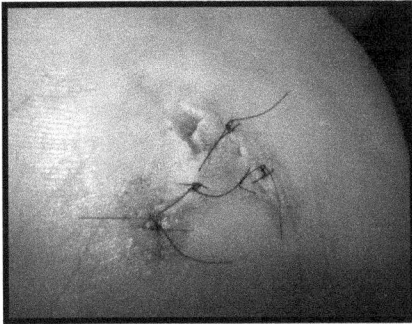

Above: suffered my biggest loss of blood when drunk classmates broke glass beer bottles during the annual "Ivies" spring music concert at Bowdoin. Pulling the glass out shot blood on my friends nearby where I lost 1 pint or 10% of my blood. This is a pain I'll always remember

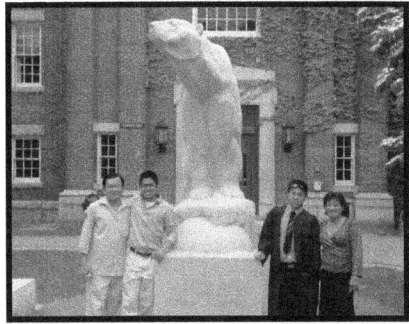

Above: made my parents proud as first in family to graduate college in America. My dad's highest was high school as he went to fight for the South Vietnamese Army and my mom's was 7th grade as she had to take care of younger siblings and help parents sell kitchenware in Vietnam

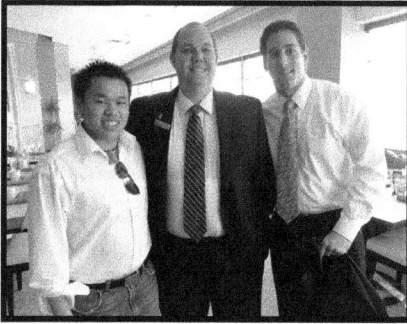

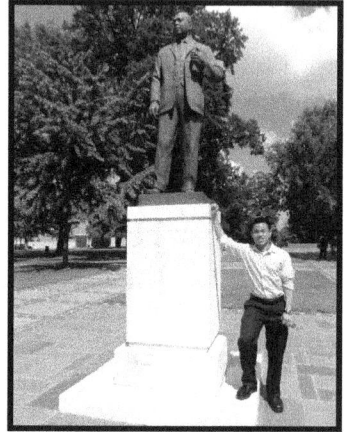

Above: first job out of college was as a management consultant where I became fat as an adult thru terrible nutrition and drinking from living in hotels 200 nights a year for 4 years straight. An unsustainable lifestyle. Reaching the highest levels for airlines and hotels is not worth being away from home

Above: visiting Dr. Martin Luther King Jr. statue in Birmingham, Alabama helped me to remind people who continue to discriminate against me and others that "nonviolence is a powerful and just weapon which cuts without wounding and ennobles the man who wields it. It is a sword that heals."

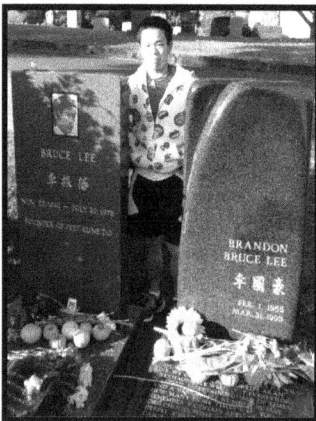

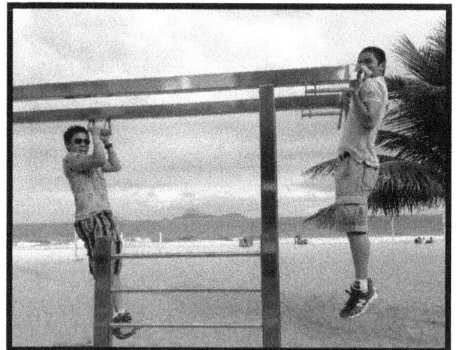

Above: during a trip to Seattle, paid respect to one of my childhood heroes Bruce Lee who paved way for martial arts to be taught to non-Asians such as he taught white Chuck Norris and black athlete Jim Kelly

Above: during a family trip to Brazil before the 2014 World Cup and 2016 Summer Olympics, exciting to see Brazil's commitment to fitness with public workout equipment. If you walk on Copacabana Beach, people from children to retirees are fit

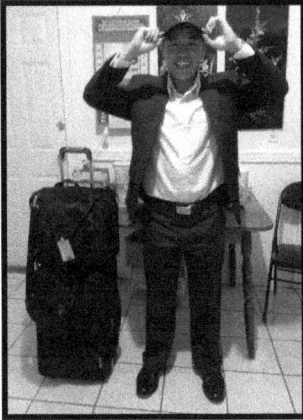

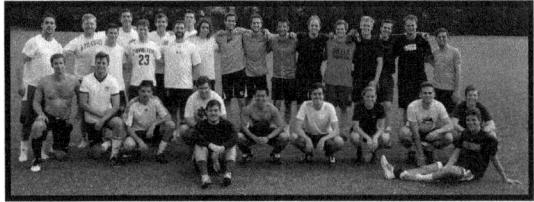

Above: wanted to make career shift from consulting to tech and entrepreneurship and also putting an end to the unhealthy lifestyle. This is my last flight as a consultant choosing Vanderbilt for MBA in Nashville, Tennessee

Above: went from fat to fit immediately by exercising at 4:44AM everyday performing 3 weight lifting and 3 martial arts workouts each week. This 2 year phase of my life changed my approach to nutrition and exercise that is the foundation for JustHuynh Fitness' method of transforming members into Ageless Athletic Assassins

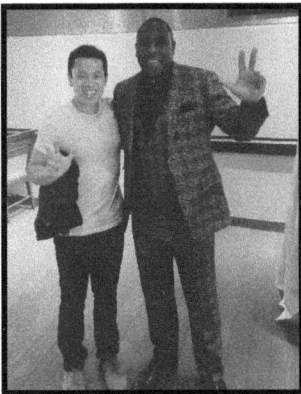

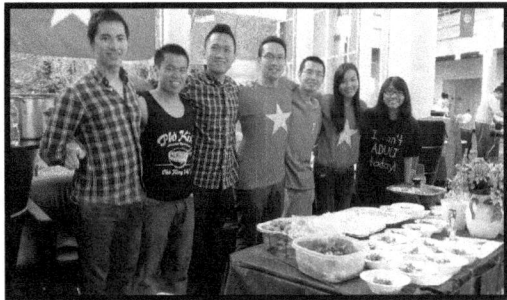

Above: proud to have chosen to attend the fittest and smartest university in the world. This is Vanderbilt Football Coach Derek Mason whose athletes I trained with at 4:44AM. I established the first annual Graduate Olympics where business school, medical school, and law school compete for fittest grads

Above: at Vanderbilt Business School's annual "Global Food Fest" where Team Vietnam is serving the national dish Pho and letting students know that by joining the "Asian Business Association" they can become stronger, sexier, and smarter

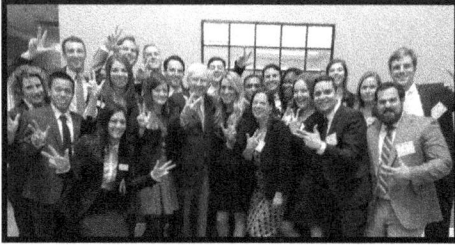

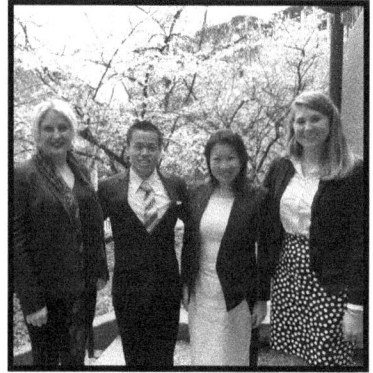

Above: Vanderbilt was invited to Warren Buffett's annual MBA day where Harvard was also in attendance with Warren mentioning that the most important thing in life for him is to have a loving and supportive wife who is there with you for the ups and downs of life

Above: Asia Business Association co-hosted with the Women's Business Association Zola CEO Shan-Lyn Ma about how to launch startups as an MBA with Zola now valued over $1 billion in the $72 billion wedding industry

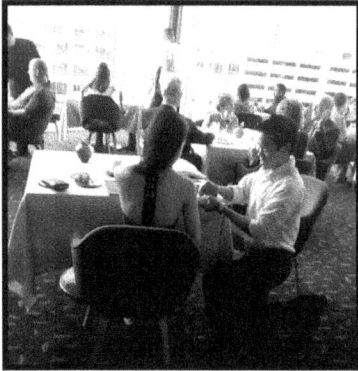

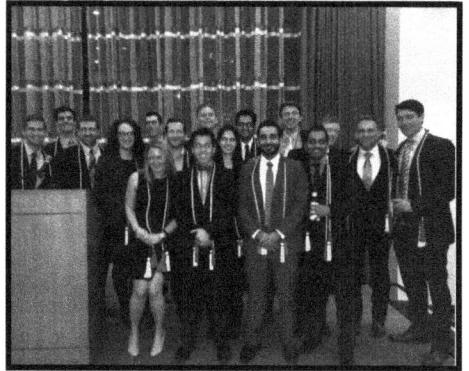

Above: biggest moment of my life as a man when I got down on my knees and proposed saying the four words "Will You Marry Me?" to my wife during her birthday at the American Restaurant in Kansas City in 2015. She said "Yes!"

Above: JustHuynh Fitness' philosophy of martial arts and power athletics have helped me thrive personally (marrying my wife), academically (Beta Gamma Sigma MBA Honor Society), athletically (fit and healthy at age 28 then), and professionally (entrepreneurial leadership)

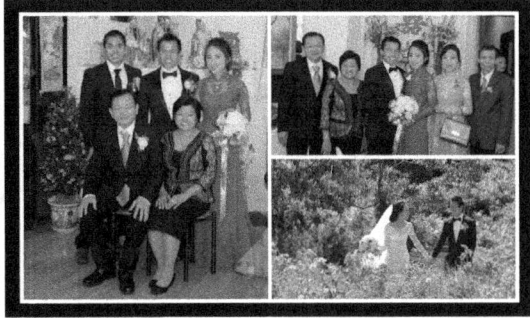

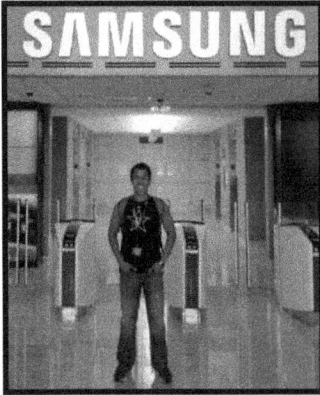

Above: my MBA internship with Samsung provided inspiration for JustHuynh Fitness to become a premium global brand that helps the over 2 billion overweight people worldwide become Ageless Athletic Assassins

Above: In 2016, my wife and I married in Vietnamese tradition driving 2 hours from Maine to Boston to pick her up for wedding in my hometown of South Portland, Maine

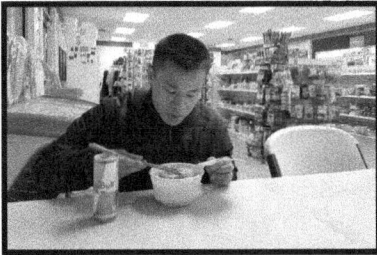

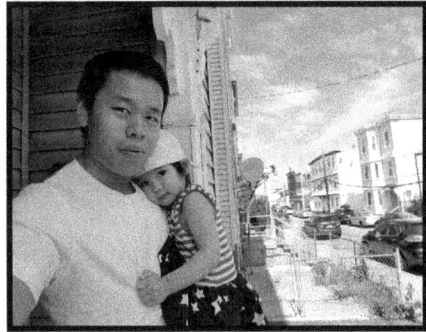

Above: with the support of my wife and parents, I rejected $100,000+ job offers from Samsung and the FBI to start from scratch launching JustHuynh Fitness. We were willing to sacrifice a high-paying job we weren't excited waking up for to pursue our calling of fitness. There are times when all I had in the bank was enough for noodles (ramen profitability)

Above: forgoing a six-figure salary also meant delaying house and having kids so this is my favorite niece Kylee who I care for as if she's my daughter since everyone is living together in Dorchester Boston until we can afford a house and have kids

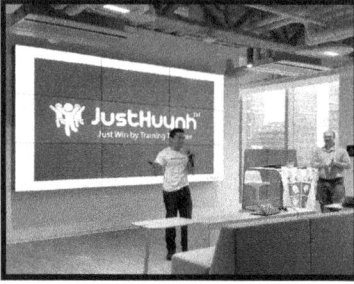

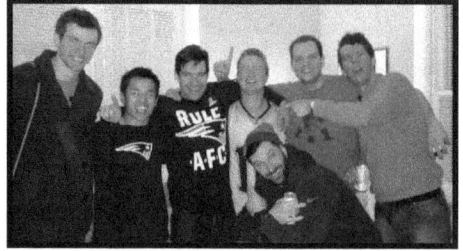

Above: JustHuynh Fitness helps people boost confidence and build self defense skills by training together online or in our fitness studio for martial arts and power athletics

Above: Born in Boston, JustHuynh Fitness cultivates a winning attitude to members so they too can "JustHuynh - Just Win" at life thru fitness like the Patriots, Red Sox, and Celtics

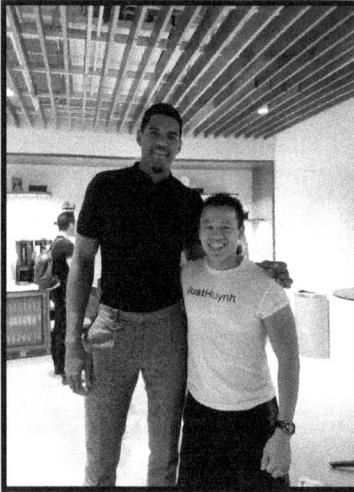

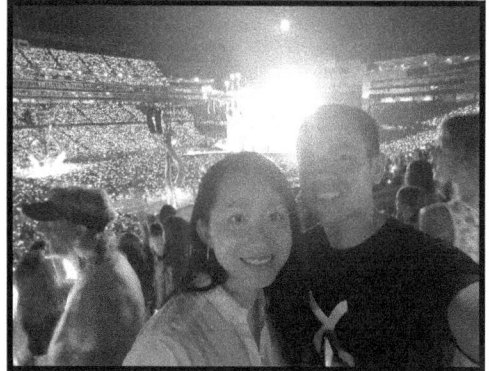

Above: Met basketball player Tobias Harris who shared about "working hard when nobody is watching" which has finally paid off for Tobias as he turned down a 4-year $80 million contract from the LA Clippers to be eligible for a max contract of 5-years $188 million ($37.6 million annual). Tobias agrees that fitness has helped him thrive personally and professionally such as with the Mamba Mentality that Kobe Bryant learnt from Bruce Lee

Above: attended and was inspired by Taylor Swift's Reputation Tour at Gillette Stadium where she performed in front of 60,000 raving fans - mostly women and girls experiencing heartbreak and love that Taylor's songs cover. As one person, Taylor impacted over 3 million fans over 53 shows that generated $345.7 million in ticket sales - the most all-time. JustHuynh Fitness hopes to inspire people to enjoy our brand of martial arts and power athletics like they do Taylor's music

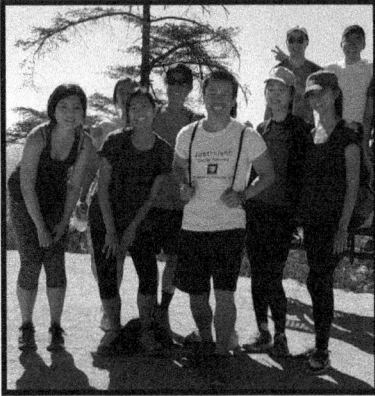

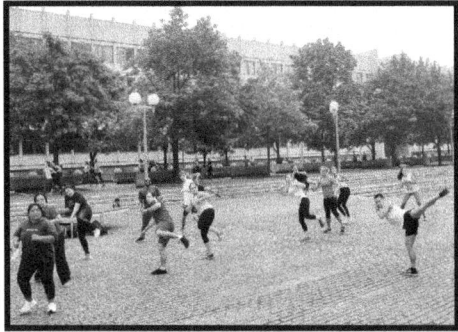

Above: JustHuynh Fitness helps UCLA college student women prevent sexual assault and men avoid bullying

Above: JustHuynh Fitness at Boston Social Fitness Festival leading community thru our signature martial arts and power athletics

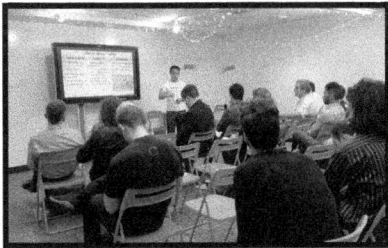

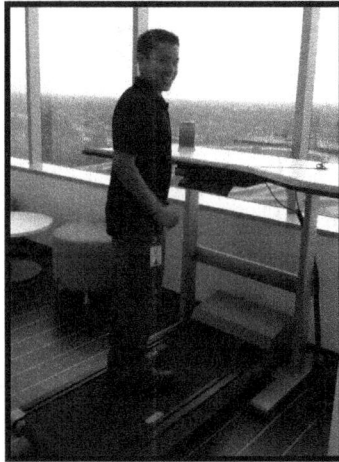

Above: JustHuynh Fitness speaking at Boston conference on "health is wealth" as too many people forget about their health when health is critical to your success in life

Above: JustHuynh Fitness' online fitness program can easily be performed at work by setting up kickboxing bags in an office area just like many companies have treadmill desks

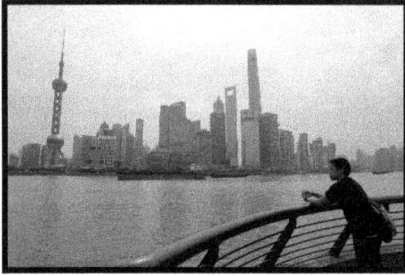

Above: first stop in 2018 Asia Tour visiting
Shanghai, China about the aspects of
Shaolin martial arts and recovery techniques
to incorporate into JustHuynh Fitness

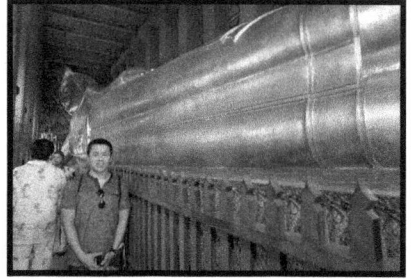

Above: second stop in 2018 Asia Tour
visiting Thailand about the aspect of Muay
Thai martial arts and benefits of massage
to incorporate into JustHuynh Fitness

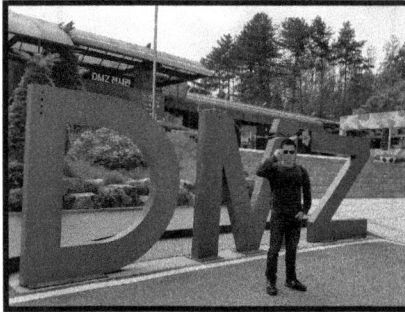

Above: third stop in 2018 Asia Tour visiting
Seoul, South Korea about the aspects of
Taekwondo martial arts and k-pop style
music to incorporate into JustHuynh Fitness

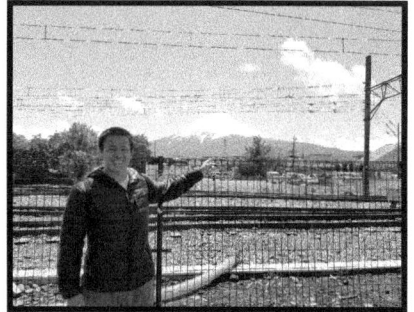

Above: fourth stop in 2018 Asia Tour visiting
Japan about the aspects of karate martial arts
and Okinawa's "land of the immortals"
Supercentenarian health habits to incorporate
into JustHuynh Fitness

CHAPTER 8

ANTI-BULLYING SELF DEFENSE

I fear not the man who has practiced 10,000 kicks once, but I fear the man who has practiced one kick 10,000 times

\- Bruce Lee

FIGHT OR FLIGHT

Out in public when you leave your house, the college bubble, workplace, or place of worship, no one cares about your prestigious college, bench press, alcohol tolerance, or net worth as its survival of the fittest. Over your lifetime, you have or are likely to encounter life-threatening situations where you need to defend yourself.

Instead of an upgrade in safety after graduating college from Maine, I moved down to Dorchester, MA where I carried a knife with me at all times wearing street clothes before changing into professional clothes when I was a consultant. There were bullet holes in my apartment mailbox and frequent shootings after the Boston Marathon bombings. Whenever someone threatening approached me, I always coughed hard to send the impression that they might catch a contagious disease. That technique kept me safe without having to use lethal physical self-defense. Back in Boston after MBA from Nashville, I drive to pick up my wife from work ever since an innocent person was shot in her car at Field's Corner station waiting for her family.

For one summer after business school, I lived in Newark New Jersey (nicknamed car theft capital of the world) where gangs killed each other after 8PM. Fortunately, I survived those living conditions due to the confidence gained with a "fight or flight" exercise regimen - garnering a nod of respect from the streets. Members of the gym would ask if I was a cop or secret agent due to my execution-style martial arts. I'd respond saying just a normal person enjoying the benefits that martial arts provides for the body and mind. No way I'd be prepared for a life threatening situation if I just "checked the box in the gym" watching TV and eating donuts during a workout. As long as I was politely working out and not causing trouble, nobody gave me trouble.

BULLIES ARE COWARDS

Bullying is one of the most cowardly acts often carried out by someone who is insecure about themselves and their only way to happiness is to pick on someone perceived to be weaker than them. These cowards wouldn't dare pick on someone who is equal or better than them.

A human's most emotional feelings arise when they're faced with a life-threatening situation. With JustHuynh Fitness' boxing and kickboxing classes, you can be street-ready for fight or flight situations in a 30 second physical confrontation or outrunning the threat in a 600 meter distance in under 100 seconds.

In elementary school, I was shy and skinny - an easy target for bullies. I never ratted as was afraid of getting beat up. At home, my parents noticed my mood and low academic performance so enrolled my brother and I in martial arts.

After 3 years of martial arts, not only did I improve physically with knowing how to punch, kick, block, dodge, and use weapons such as the bo staff, I improved my confidence and academic performance - getting admitted into an elite liberal arts college (Bowdoin College) and MBA Program (Vanderbilt University).

Living in one town during my grade school years, those same bullies from elementary school also attended the same middle school. One day during 8th grade history class, these same bullies decided to bully me into proving my martial arts skills as I was now fitter and smarter than them. In martial arts, we learn for health and self-defense - never to attack. Conveniently, our 8th grade history teacher was a former soldier so gave me the "nod" to carry out my self-defense training. When one of the bullies grabbed my hand, I responded by twisting his wrist and dragged him across the classroom demanding him to tell the entire class that he would never again bully. The bully gave us his word and classmates respected how much martial arts can improve one physically and mentally.

Like Bruce Lee said, you should fear someone who has practiced a particular move at least 10,000 times well. An average martial arts class involved perfecting a move 100 times. Having gone to classes 6 times a week, it would take 17 weeks to cover the 100 needed classes for move mastery.

My favorite moves are the shuffle-side kick and rib cage body shot as they are both powerful and can be quickly executed. With so much practice and sparring, these moves were now mind to muscle memory with instant reaction based on the incoming stimuli.

Martial arts practitioners hope to never use their self-defense in public, but must if our lives are in danger. As the only Vietnamese/Chinese person in my class, my parents took us on a family trip to New York City with a stop in Chinatown to see Asian culture in a large city. With over 1 million Chinese Americans in New York City's Chinatown, we were overwhelmed coming from our tiny town of South Portland, Maine with 25,000 residents.

While shopping, my parents left my brother and I in the public playground - maintaining eyes on us. As my brother was playing with his new toy, 5 bigger and taller boys came out of nowhere with one of the boys throwing an uppercut punch to my brother's gut causing him to drop the toy for them to take. With my innocent brother hurting due to bullying, I had to defend my brother before further damage was inflicted to him.

Five against two, this was the first time in my life that I had to unleash my self defense martial arts to protect our lives. I immediately went after the guy standing over my brother with my most powerful kick - the shuffle side kick that dropped him to the ground in pain. This first guy turned out to be the leader so when the next two guys came up, I fired a right rib-cage shot to the guy on the left - dropping him then performed a wrist twist on the third guy making him kneel on the ground. As typical in most fights, the other two ran away. With all three guys down, I told them to stop the bullying, picked up my injured brother, and went back to find our parents.

Full of emotion, we told our parents about the bullying when my dad was proud of how we handled the bullying situation. My dad let us know that a travelling adult friend had asked "who's the boy who just sidekicked the other boy to the ground?" When my dad said that was his son - me, and that I could handle it, he was indeed proud that we safely executed our self-defense training to protect our lives from bullying.

Children experience bullying all the time. When it gets physical in public, self-defense can help children avoid getting hurt by bigger bullies.

SEXUAL ASSAULT & #METOO

Whether male or female, both genders are susceptible to sexual assault and it's awful when we experience the feeling of helplessness.

Before learning martial arts, I experienced a horrific sexual assault during my childhood that I will always remember. This was in Vung Tau Beach in Vietnam for family vacation. As I sat on the beach half-naked quietly playing with sand with no family members within speaking distance, a random adult man comes by to squeeze and slap my boob. Being fat at this point in life, the man creepily loved that my boob shook back and forth like Jell-O. Shy and unable to defend myself, I didn't do anything so this sexual assault moment is forever ingrained in my brain. As an adult now, my only wish is for karma to strike back at this disgusting man.

I'm not the only young boy falling victim to sexual assault as you see stories of priests sexually molesting church boys. In 2018, the Pennsylvania Supreme Court in the United States revealed that 300 Catholic Priests sexually abused 1,000 children. 17 years earlier in 2001, the Boston Globe's Spotlight team uncovered that 6% of Boston's Catholic Priests (91) sexually abused children with 50% of priests not celibate. This is documented in the 2015 movie "Spotlight." If sexual abuse can occur and have cover-up attempts in the most sacred and powerful institution such as the church, we should all be concerned as parents who send our children - especially boys to religious study without parental supervision.

High school girls and college women are susceptible to sexual assault especially rape. When I was in grade school and college, there wasn't self defense resources for females. Today in 2018, I was happy to hear that my cousin in high school is provided Wing-Chun training once a week from her school's resource officer and from my cousin who attends a college that requires two years of mandatory exercise classes. She's currently taking yoga, but hopefully the school will offer self-defense classes.

Now on how college sports programs impact campus safety.

Countries love football otherwise known as soccer in America as evident by the patriotism exhibited every four years at the World Cup. Soccer is a sport anyone can simply play barefoot by kicking a ball between a couple rocks or trash can. In America, American football and basketball are the most popular sports with stars well-known all over the world. Colleges and universities serve as a pipeline for professional talent with the most successful sports programs getting a boost in college applications and more importantly alumni donations that fuel the school's endowments. Schools thrive when basketball and football athletes succeed in tournament play as a "winning" culture brings positivity to a school's social life and prideful alumni who brag to their co-workers by happily donating a larger than normal amount.

In college basketball, success in the annual tournament of 64 teams called "March Madness" can change a school's status instantly that originated in 1984 when Boston College (BC) quarterback Doug Flutie's "Hail Mary" pass at the 1984 Orange Bowl dethroned defending national champion University of Miami. Following the epic victory, Boston College saw applications increase by 30%, boost in alumni giving, and rose to #32 ranked best university in the United States. Any college experiencing such boost in applications, alumni giving, and ranking increase from sports victories achieves what's now called "The Flutie Effect" in honor of Doug Flutie's game changing play. A recent basketball example is when unknown UMBC achieved the greatest upset in college basketball history by defeating #1 ranked University of Virginia as a #16 rank with a 5,000-to-1 odds in Las Vegas' sportsbook. Overwhelmed by instant alumni donations and college applications, the surge in online traffic crashed the school's website server. At University of Connecticut (UConn), women's basketball head coach Geno Auriemma has led the university to 11 NCAA Division 1 national championships from 1995-2018. The championships brought in billions of dollars in public funds and alumni donations to upgrade UConn's academic infrastructure and school's stature. After Geno won his first title for UConn in 1995, he visited the state legislature who voted to pump $1 billion into "UConn 2000" campus improvement project.

Although high school recruits and players on the University of Louisville's basketball team did not initiate sexual assault, they engaged in sex parties organized by director of basketball operations Andre McGee under head Coach Rick Pitino. From 2010-2014 with the team winning the NCAA Division 1 national championship in 2013, Andre McGee paid escort Katina Powell $10,000 to organize 22 sex parties in dorm rooms of which 20 prospects and student-athletes participated. For violating NCAA policy, Louisville vacated its 2013 Championship Title and repaid shared NCAA tournament revenue from the 2012-2015 appearances. It is disturbing that Louisville promoted a culture where young high-school boys and college students participate in sex acts in exchange for playing time. These students may be susceptible to sexually assaulting women as adults.

A winning football program touches the entire student life-cycle from television awareness, better social life, alumni return for "homecoming" games, and more alumni donation for pride in the school's football success. With football and basketball dominating life at more than 5,000 universities in America, sexual assault by these athletes still occurs.

At Baylor University, 22-year old Tevin Elliott was sentenced to 20 years in state prison for 2 rape charges against a female Baylor athlete. What's shocking is that Baylor University and football head coach Art Briles were aware of Tevin's assault but covered up its student reports to boost the school's status and alumni giving. During Art Briles' coaching tenure, a lawsuit cited that at least 31 football players committed 52 rapes where some were gang raped by 5 football players at once. Art Briles was fired.

Males are also at-risk of sexual assault when former Ohio State team doctor Richard Strauss was accused by over 100 former Ohio State students that the doctor abused them from 1979-1997. The former male victims came from 14 sports (baseball, cheerleading, cross country, fencing, football, gymnastics, ice hockey, lacrosse, soccer, swimming, tennis, track, volleyball and wrestling). Although Richard Strauss committed suicide in 2005, the investigation is seeing if any Ohio State personnel failed to stop Richard from performing the sexual assaults.

At Florida State University (FSU) Erica Kinsman sued FSU for mishandling her alleged rape by Heisman Trophy-winning quarterback Jameis Winston when Jameis took her clothes off in his apartment and engaged in intercourse despite her objections. FSU settled $950,000 with Erica and attorneys. After being drafted #1 overall in the 2015 NFL Draft, Jameis Winston still hasn't learned to respect women by groping a female Uber driver in inappropriate parts without her consent - he was suspended 3 games.

As a rising or current college student, alumni, or future college parent, it is important to be aware about sexual assault dangers by male athletes who think they are above the law. Head coaches and administrators tend to cover up sexual assault allegations by quietly paying off victims. College girls or boys equipped with self-defense techniques can fight off assaults.

As adults, women may face sexual assault at work or could be kidnapped into sex trafficking. Men in prison, all-male clubs, or small businesses are likely targets of sexual abuse. With #metoo at its height from April 2017-November 2018, there have been 252 celebrities, politicians, CEOs, and others accused of sexual misconduct per Vox. The list is long with the purpose that sexual assault occurs towards any gender and age. In sports, Larry Nassar was sentenced to 40-175 years in prison for sexually assaulting over 160 women - mostly gymnasts. In entertainment, Harvey Weinstein was accused by more than 80 women for sexual assault, Asia Argento was accused of assaulting a 17 year old boy when she was 37, Allison Mack recruited 150 women to join a sex-cult - branding them as slaves, Bill Cosby was sentenced 3-10 years in prison for sexually assaulting 60 women, Louis C.K. stripped naked and masturbated in front of 5 women without their consent, and Kevin Spacey was accused by 15 men - including five teens at the time, that he sexually assaulted them. In media, former CBS CEO Leslie Moonves forced former actress Bobbie Phillips to give him oral sex in exchange for a role in a TV show, Bill O'Reilly of Fox News settled a sexual harassment claim for $32 million with Lis Wiehl, 20-year "Today" Show host Matt Lauer was accused of sexually assaulting an employee until she passed out and had to be taken to a nurse, and Kimberly Guilfoyle - single-mom and girlfriend of recently divorced Donald Trump Jr., was accused of showing colleagues personal photographs of male genitalia and discussing sexual matters at work. In tech, investors Shervin Pishevar, former "Shark Tank" investor Chris Sacca, Dave McClure, Justin Caldbeck, and former Uber CEO Travis Kalanick were all accused of sexual assault.

Here are some real life examples when self-defense training saved a man or woman's life.

In 2018 in Boston, Ebrahim Gawargi a 5 feet 7 inch man weighing 120 pounds was working as a cashier at a gas station on a Tuesday night when a robber came out of nowhere trying to take $600 from the cash register. What the robber didn't know was that Ebrahim trained four hours a day in martial arts over the past two years so had to apply self-defense for the first time such as I did in New York City by throwing a couple punches for the attacker to fall then put him to sleep with a rear-naked choke before calling the police. Another example of how martial arts can save your life.

In 2017, Kelly Herron was jogging in Seattle on Sunday and decided to use a public restroom but was shocked when she turned around to see a man standing behind her in the bathroom. Kelly mentioned that the sex offender took her to the ground by hitting her knees and legs. Having taken a 2 hour self-defense class, she escaped by clawing his face. We must be careful about outside surroundings as a sexual offender could always be lurking around waiting to attack when you're least likely to expect an attack coming.

In 2017, real estate agent Sherri Hinkel of Nebraska was showing a home to a potential home buyer who creepily invited her to the master bedroom where he took down his shorts and touched himself asking Sherri to get in bed with him. Sherri mentioned that her martial arts training provided her the ability to notice that the creepy man was acting weird by asking her to enter the master bedroom first so he could trap her in the room with him had she gone first. Fortunately she called the cops ahead of time to avoid being sexually assaulted. Service businesses that involve person to person interactions are potential opportunities for sexual predators. In the real estate industry where agents show empty properties to prospective clients, safety is a major issue. According to the National Association of Realtors, 25% of male and 12% of female realtors carry a gun. Many also download a safety app and carry pepper spray or a taser. When dealing one on one, turn your self-defense radar on.

Other industries susceptible to sexual predators is ride-sharing (Uber, Lyft), home-sharing (AirBnB), dog-walking (Wag), massages (Soothe), non-martial arts fitness instructors (ClassPass), babysitters (care.com, urbansitter), dating (Tinder, Bumble, Seeking Arrangement), in-home maintenance (handy, taskrabbit), etc.

DAILY PRACTICE - 10,000 REPS

Like Bruce Lee mentioned, perfecting the execution of particular martial arts self-defense techniques 10,000 times will allow you to react naturally to neutralize threats.

Hollywood actors know the value of commitment. In training for the filming of "Kill Bill" - a movie about a woman who trained in martial arts to avenge the death of her child, Uma Thurman, Lucy Liu, Daryl Hannah, David Carradine, and Vivica Fox spent eight hours a day (9AM-5PM Monday through Friday) for 3 months studying martial arts. That's Olympic Level commitment - resulting in a terrific film and boosted self-defense life skills.

JustHuynh Fitness prepares you for fight (self-defense thru martial arts and weight lifting) or flight (speedy escape thru sprinting) skills against threats. You should be able to last in a fight for 30 seconds or outrun your opponent in 100 seconds.

When exercising embrace the mindset of a fighter, world-class athlete, or CEO preparing to defeat the competition. Personally, I have a motivation wall to channel my inner Bruce Lee and Super Saiyan when working out. You can create your own motivation wall with your favorite martial artists or super heros.

Don't be the person with the big bench who can't run up a flight of stairs? Or don't be the person who can run 10 miles on the treadmill but who can't help someone move a couch? By giving just 4.44% of your time for 110% results, you can be the best strength and conditioned "Ageless Athletic Assassin" pound for pound ready for fight or flight situations.

CHAPTER 9

SUPERHUMAN WARRIOR SKILLS

What counts is not necessarily the size of the dog in the fight - it's the size of the fight in the dog

- President Dwight D. Eisenhower

SUPERMAN & WONDERWOMAN

Growing up many of us dreamed of becoming a superhero. For females it may be Wonder Woman starring Gal Gadot, Beatrix from "Kill Bill" starring Uma Thurman or Riley North in "Peppermint" starring Jennifer Garner. Males love Superman, Batman, Spiderman, James Bond, John Wick starring Keanu Reeves, Jack Reacher or Ethan Hunt starring Tom Cruise, or Jason Bourne starring Matt Damon.

Bill in "Kill Bill" has a great line about superheroes saying "An essential characteristic of the superhero mythology is there's the superhero and there's the alter ego. Batman is actually Bruce Wayne. Spider-Man is actually Peter Parker. When Spider-Man wakes up in the morning, he's Peter Parker. He has to put on a costume to become Spider-Man. And it is in that characteristic that Superman stands alone. Superman did not become Superman, Superman was born Superman. When Superman wakes up in the morning, he's Superman. His alter ego is Clark Kent. His outfit with the big red "S" as a baby when the Kents found him. Those are his clothes. The glasses, the business suit - that's the costume Superman wears to blend in with us. Clark Kent is how Superman views us. He's weak, he's unsure of himself... he's a coward. Clark Kent is Superman's critique on the whole human race."

At JustHuynh Fitness, our mission is to improve your confidence and self-defense skills so you too can channel your inner Superman or Wonder Woman as needed.

ARTIFICIAL VS HUMAN INTELLIGENCE

We all survived the moment we became an embryo when 1 of your father's 200 million sperm won the battle to match with your mother's egg to create you. The odds of you making the right decision to exercise (50%) are better than odds of 1/200 million sperm that created you. As Yoda from "Star Wars" says "Do or do not. There is no try." The more you delay prioritizing your fitness, the earlier you'll be susceptible to health issues such as obesity, diabetes, cancer, and even death.

After the passing of Apple's Steve Jobs, Tesla's Elon Musk is now considered the most innovative person in the world working on electric cars, space rockets, solar panels, speed tunnels, artificial intelligence, and much more. Similar to how human intelligence and physical capabilities helped our species overpower other animals, Elon fears that artificial intelligence will inevitably exceed human intelligence thus turning humans into endangered species where humans will be driven into small pockets of existence such as being displayed in the zoo.

Movies such as "The Terminator," "Her," "Wall-E,""The Matrix," "Blade Runner 2049," "Resident Evil," "Passengers," "Tron," "RoboCop," "Star Wars," "Star Trek" and TV shows such as "Westworld" all depict a world dominated by artificial intelligence. Elon has gone on record saying it may be wise for humans to join forces with artificial intelligence to appease artificial intelligence about any thoughts of eliminating the human race.

SUPER SOLDIERS - WORLD WAR III

Countries around the world especially the United States, China, and Russia are investing billions of dollars into research on creating physically and mentally strong super soldiers to be the strongest fighters on Earth. The rise of artificial intelligence, virtual reality, anti-ageing DNA research, and human cloning can lead to an army of genetic super soldiers. As a "Street Fighter" fan growing up, a scenario where world powers such as the U.S., China, or Russia take over the world with super soldiers is eerily similar to the plotline where General M. Bison conquered the world with an army of genetic super soldiers who defeated the protagonist Allied Nations. A world where one leader dominates the world with an army of super soldiers is actually within reach as at the 2017 19th World Festival of Youth and Students in Sochi Russia, Russian leader Vladimir Putin warned that scientists will be able to create an army of genetically engineered soldiers that will not feel "fear, compassion, regret, or pain" saying "What I have just described might be worse than a nuclear bomb. Whatever we do, we must never forget about the ethical foundations of our work." Super soldiers will be humans immersed in artificial intelligence with Putin saying "Artificial intelligence is the future, not only for Russia, but for all humankind. Whoever becomes the leader in this sphere will become the ruler of the world." Elon Musk concurs with Putin on Twitter tweeting "China, Russia, soon all countries with strong computer science. Competition for AI superiority at national level most likely cause of WW3."

In the United States, the Defense Advanced Research Projects Agency (DARPA) is an agency of the United States Department of Defense responsible for the development of emerging technologies for use by the military. There are many emerging technologies being developed for super soldiers including software that can be uploaded directly to the brain that heightens a soldier's senses while also curing ailments such as blindness, paralysis, and speech disorders; a contact lens that improves vision tenfold, an exoskeleton called XOS 2 developed by Raytheon that makes soldiers 17 times stronger such as being able to carry 400 pounds but only feeling the weight of 23.53 pounds, bulletproof clothes made of carbon graphene chainmail developed by MIT's Institute for Soldier Nanotechnologies, synthetic blood cells called respirocyte where soldiers will never run out of breath and can spend hours underwater without breathing equipment; bionic boots that mimic kangaroo tendons to augment the human ankle and Achilles tendon that will allow soldiers to jump seven feet high, sprint at inhuman speed faster than Olympic champions, and run all day without wearing out muscles; pain immunizations where soldiers won't feel pain while in battle gives them 30 days to fight without feeling serious pain and regrow limbs lost in combat; sleep freedom similar to that experienced by ENU mice who are nocturnal without needing sleep; telepathy powers where soldiers can control robots with their thoughts and communicate with other soldiers using their minds; gecko-like climbing gloves and shoes to go up skyscrapers; squirrel gene that allows humans to conserve energy via hibernation in cold winter conditions; neurostimulation to accelerate learning; super-strong immune system; hunger-free to go for days without food, and soldiers will have their empathy genes deleted that allow them to show no mercy and no fear.

SWIMMING - MICHAEL PHELPS

The NAVY SEALS acronym stands for sea, air, and land. Along with sprinting (land) and fighting (air), swimming is one of the best cardio exercises. It's the sea portion of my personal NAVY SEALS fitness approach.

Swimming provides many life benefits such as boosting youthfulness, weight loss, and intelligence.

To be in the right mindset, it helps to use inspiration and motivation so that you complete your swimming workouts strong. For inspiration, I personally use Michael Phelps as a mindset to strive for as he's always focused in tuning out distractions to win Olympic Gold medals such as his 8 gold medals at the 2008 Beijing Olympics.

For motivation, there will be times when you might not have enough endurance in the deep section of the pool that could result in drowning. I never took swimming lessons, but learned how to swim thru drowning at Age 10 being rescued by the lifeguard at a public swimming pool. Since that moment instead of fearing swimming, I motivated myself that I must survive to help people become healthier thru martial arts and power athletics. Today, the internal motivation I use is that I need to finish the swim without drowning in order to save my wife in a dangerous part of the ocean. This visual pops in my mind every time my body might give up in the deep section of the pool or open water.

Now with your mindset right, let's go over the benefits.

Weight loss: Water is denser than air so moving through H2O puts more external pressure on your limbs than out-of-water training. People who consistently swim to be out of breath burn calories and lose weight.

Anti-ageing: Regular swimmers are biologically 20 years younger than their driver's licenses say they are. At the age of 30, officers and bouncers think I'm 18 years old sporting a fake ID.

Intelligence: Blood flow to the brain increased up to 14 percent when men and women submerged themselves in water up to their hearts, according to a Journal of Physiology study. Researchers believe water's pressure on the chest cavity provides the increased blood flow to brain.

Physique: Swimming fires up more of your body's major muscle groups than other forms of cardio exercise. When you're running or biking, you're mostly using your lower body. Swimming not only engages your legs, but also involves your upper body and core for a beach body look.

Speed and endurance: By increasing your ability to take in and effectively use oxygen, swimming increases your endurance capacity allowing you to run faster on land without getting winded.

Stress reducer: Being submerged in water dulls the amount of sensory information that bombards your body helping you feel calm

SPRINTING - USAIN BOLT

Sprinting is one of the best cardio exercises. It's the land portion of my personal NAVY SEALS fitness approach. Sprinting provides many life benefits such as mental toughness, weight loss, and physique. Many people are obsessed with speed for fast people (Usain Bolt is the fastest person ever running 100 meters in 8.70 seconds which is 41 km/h or 25.48 mph), fast horses (In 2008, Winning Brew covered 402 meters in 20.57 seconds which is 70.76 km/h or 43.97 mph. What's interesting is that horses are worth more when they're retired due to the strong offspring produced. America's most valuable horse 'Tapit' makes $300,000 every time he has sex to give birth called a "stud fee" which he can do 135 times a year for the next 10 years that nets his owners $40 million a year), fast cars (The Hennessey Venom F5, which cost $1.6 million, goes at 301 mph with ability to accelerate to 249 mph and brake down to a full stop in under 30 seconds with 1,600 horsepower), and fast planes (The North American X-15, which cost $9 million in 1964, is the fastest plane in the world at Mach 6.70 which is 7,200 km/h or 4,474 mph. Mach 1 or 768 mph is the speed of sound otherwise known as supersonic speed).

To be in the right mindset, it helps to use inspiration and motivation so that you complete your sprinting workouts when you're out of breath or the lactic acid kicks in. For inspiration, I personally use Usain Bolt as a mindset to strive for as he always comes out of the blocks slow, but has amazing closing speed to win the 100 meter Olympic Gold Medal.

For motivation, there will be times when you feel like not finishing your sprinting session due to boredom, lack of motivation, or fatigue. As a 5'2" guy, I've always been discriminated for being short and unathletic because I'm Asian so most people only come to me for math questions. Fortunately for others, I don't go protesting, but instead help educate the discriminators on how to treat everyone with respect regardless of their race, age, or physique either thru a humble athletic beatdown or cultural education.

During business school, one of my classmates challenged me to a 300 meter sprint and was 100 percent confident he'd win because I was short and

Asian compared to him who was 5'8' and a former wrestler. Not knowing his actual speed, I took the challenge and we agreed that the loser would donate money to the Wounded Warriors project. It was a huge business school spectacle with the entire school watching where I finished in 42 seconds and the classmate lost by 18 seconds - with onlookers begging for mercy near the end of the race. We shook hands and he has respected me ever since. I even invited him to my Bachelor Party in Iceland and Wedding in Maine!

I've always thrived on being an underdog with a chip on my shoulder. For every single sprint, this challenge by my classmate and coming behind to win the race as anchor of a track relay against competitors much younger than I, puts me in a winning mindset. If this is not enough, I visualize that I have to catch a criminal who can only survive if they can sprint for more than 52 seconds. Now with your mindset right, let's go over the benefits.

Mental toughness: Sprints are a challenging workout. There may be moments where you want to quit. Pushing through the negative thoughts will build confidence in your emotional and physical abilities.

Reduce Stress: Sprinting produces endorphins which are chemicals in the brain that act as natural painkillers and provide you with a "feel good" sensation from any stresses.

Heart Rate: As you sprint, your heart rate increases to compensate for the increased need for blood flow to your sprinting muscles. Over time, sprint training increases your maximum heart rate and cardiovascular fitness.

Anaerobic Threshold: Sprinting is an anaerobic exercise that requires short bursts of energy producing lactic acid. The buildup of lactic acid leads to pain and soreness. With more sprint reps, your anaerobic threshold will rise allowing you to be faster and stronger.

Metabolism: Sprinting burns a great deal of calories in short amount of time compared with slower long distance running. As a high intensity form of exercise, sprinting boosts the body's metabolism that helps prevent weight gain and diabetes. You'll also benefit from the afterburn effect 24-48 hours after exercises where you burn more calories after your exercise.

Physique: When weight training, your body is required to produce short bursts of energy that increase muscle strength. Sprinting works in the same way. However, unlike weightlifting, sprinting uses dozens of muscles at the same time, making it a full body muscle training. A study conducted in 2012 showed sprinting can enhance protein synthesis pathways by as much as 230 percent! With the right nutrition and recovery, this will lead to muscle building, allowing your body to become leaner and enabling you to run faster, longer, and more efficiently.

SELF DEFENSE - BRUCE LEE

Self defense consisting of kickboxing, karate, and kungfu is one of the best cardio exercises. It's the air portion of my personal NAVY SEALS fitness approach. Martial arts provides many life benefits such as confidence, weight loss, physique, and self defense. With the popularity of mixed martial arts competitions, celebrities ranging from models to actors to business executives realize that martial arts is the best fat burning and healthy form of cardio.

To be in the right mindset, it helps to use inspiration and motivation so that you complete your martial arts workouts when you're tired. For inspiration, I use Bruce Lee as a mindset who took his training to the highest level being respected by martial art legends like Chuck Norris and Asian martial artists from karate, kung-fu, taekwondo, and muay thai. Such a tragedy that a legend like Bruce Lee died so young at Age 32 back in 1973 and still leaves a lasting legacy on action stars and aspiring martial artists.

For motivation, there will be times when you feel winded with no more leg or arm power. My all-time favorite match was when I defeated a 3rd degree black belt with only 9 months of karate experience. At the time, I was at a huge disadvantage experience wise, but wanted to test my self defense from watching Bruce Lee and Chinese Kung Fu films. In front of my dojo, I shocked everyone by winning the sparring fight by baiting the black belt to throw a front kick in which I ducked down for a left leg sweep that tripped them up and followed with a flying right front kick to their stomach when they were mid-air to win the point. The sensei immediately halted the match and asked where I learned that technique because that wasn't karate. I mentioned from Chinese Kung Fu movies which impressed the sensei.

In addition to the memorable fight, I channel my Dragon Ball-Z anger to take my sessions to another level as if I had to kill a villain to save the world. In the fitness industry, the enemy is anyone a part of the sickness industry such as ineffective weight loss scams, fad diet programs, time-killers, fast food, and alcohol that enable people to become overweight. Now with your mindset right, let's go over the benefits.

Weight Loss: A one hour session of moderate intensity martial arts can burn up to 500 calories. As a full body workout, your stamina, muscle tone, flexibility, reflexes, balance, and strength will all improve through martial arts. Your improved metabolism will help prevent obesity as you'll burn more calories each day thru the afterburn effect.

Self Defense: The ability to defend yourself against an assailant with speed and power is an empowering feeling.

Cognitive improvements: A 2016 study in the Journal of Sport and Health Science suggest that martial arts specific blend of aerobics, balance, and coordination provide benefits to the brain making you smarter. Continual practicing of self defense techniques until the moves become second nature improves your muscle memory. In 1999 the city of Naperville, Illinois required all 19,000 8th grade students to enroll in gym class. With 30% of 8th grade students in the United States overweight, Naperville, IL's 8th graders were one of the fittest in the United States with only 3% of students overweight. In addition to exercise transforming their bodies, exercise also strengthened the mind as evidenced after the 8th graders took the TIMSS (Trends in International Mathematics and Science Study) against powerhouses China, Japan, and Singapore. Naperville's 8th graders scored 1st in science and 6th in math all thanks to fitness. This study is further detailed in John Ratey's "Spark" book if you'd like to read more.

Confidence: With your ability to complete tough martial arts workouts, you can accomplish anything you set your mind to.

Better mood: Participating in martial arts is one of the best ways to improve your mood as exercise produces endorphins which are chemicals in the brain that act as natural painkillers and provide you with a "feel good" sensation from any stresses going on in your life.

HUMAN ANATOMY KILL SHOTS

In the streets when you need to defend yourself, you typically need to be able to defeat your opponent in under 30 seconds or be able to outrun them within 100 seconds to get to safety. According to the FBI's 2017 Crime Clock in the United States, a violent crime occurs every 24.6 seconds, one murder every 30.5 minutes, one rape every 3.9 minutes, one robbery every 1.7 minutes, and one aggravated assault every 39 seconds so it's extremely important you can run, hide, or defend yourself.

Similar to Bruce Lee being able to knock out opponents with his "One Inch Punch," military snipers adopt a "One Shot, One Kill" philosophy by being efficient in taking down a threat in as little time and energy spent as possible. In a life threatening situation, your knowledge of the human anatomy will allow you to take down the threat quickly so you can escape danger. Below are parts of the body (top to bottom) that you can practice with a padded person, dummy, or shadow boxing to defend yourself. These parts of the body have been identified as pressure points in acupuncture that will bring pain to the attacker. We live in an age where anyone can attack us in public including people you know so you must be ready to defend at all times. Use your judgment on which body parts to strike based on the threat level.

For fighting stance, you want to have a compact stance with feet directly under your shoulder where you are loose and relaxed yet springy and coiled. Keep your rear heel raised so can react like a coiled spring for kicks, punches, dodges, blocks, and other moves. For efficiency, use your hands for upper body targets and legs for lower body targets.

In practice, use a peripheral vision drill where you don't concentrate too hard on one area of the opponent but instead look at the center of opponent's body so you have peripheral vision of their entire body. Speedy reaction time involves understanding your opponent's intent of attack, retreat, punch, or kick that triggers you to evade, block, intercept, or counter. Through practice, you'll be able to relay your opponent's stimulus to your brain that triggers your self defense. You also need to be able to strike and adjust quickly in case the opponent sets you up for a counter.

Center of skull on top of head: you can break opponent's skull once they are on the ground. If you watch Hong Kong movies featuring Bak Mei, one of the five legendary Shaolin elders, opponents try to attack his groin as its perceived to be his "weak spot." When they fail, Bak Mei always kills them with the downward palm strike to the center of their skull. You can also use a flying downward elbow strike.

Temple: a strong punch to a soft temple can knock someone unconscious. You can strike with elbows, knuckle punches, and palm strikes.

Eyes: gouging an attacker in the eyes is a last resort as it can permanently damage an attacker's vision. You can use a finger jab where you tuck your long fingers to match length of pinky and tuck thumb in to form a spear. Thrust your fingers forward without retraction like a snake.

Nose: it only takes seven pounds of pressure to break a nose. Use an upward palm strike that hits bottom of the nose.

Jaw hinge: knocking someone just below the ear can break their jaw and knock them out. Your hand might get hurt as you don't have gloves like a boxer so use your palm or elbows.

Chin: striking someone on the chin can knock someone out because it forces the head to twist and rattle the brain. You can do upward palm strike, upward elbow, or flying knee strike. You can see when Jackie Chan finishes Benny Urquidez with a flying knee strike to the chin in "Wheels on Meals."

Base of skull/neck: hitting someone at the base of the skull can cause spinal cord injuries. You can strike with the bottom of your fist or use an inward elbow.

Side of neck: striking the carotid artery can cause severe dizziness. This can be executed with an open-hand karate chop.

Base of throat: a light punch to the throat can cause someone to choke. You can use a palm strike or punch. In "Mission: Impossible - Fallout," Liang Yang causes Henry Cavill to lose his breathe in the famous bathroom fight scene with Tom Cruise. Liang overpowered both men and was only defeated by getting shot.

Clavicle: this is a pressure point that can be pressed down on from behind an attacker.

Solar plexus: a strong kick or punch to the solar plexus will easily knock the wind out of someone.

Wrist: this is a pressure point where you can break an attacker's wrist by twisting the wrist outwards to drop them.

Central area of the forearm: located 5 inches before the wrist, you can intercept a punch and apply pressure on the tendons.

Behind elbow: this is the location of the funny bone that can be struck with counter elbow or punch. In the movie "Kill Zone 2," Wu Jing decapitates Zhang Chi by twisting his wrist then snapping his elbow.

Biceps: attacker will be unable to move arm if you hit their biceps so you can use this time to perform a rear naked choke hold. In "IP Man 2," Donnie Yen defeats Twister by elbow striking Twister's biceps.

Fists: when an attacker throws a jab or reverse punch, you can counter with an elbow strike that intercepts their punch. If your elbow is well conditioned, you could break the attacker's hand.

Bottom of rib cage: causes serious lesions to chest and internal organs. You can use a body shot punch or knees. You can see this being carried out by Mad Dog when he fights against Rama (Iko Uwais) and Andi in the movie "The Raid Redemption."

Liver: a strike to the right side of the rib cage can incapacitate a person. You can use a left roundhouse kick or left body punch.

Tailbone: a strong strike can send pain to rear end, lower back, and legs. You can perform a front kick.

Groin: if someone is coming at you from the front, a groin kick may deliver enough force to paralyze your attacker. In the movie "The Protectors" final fight scene, Tony Jaa escapes from a choke hold against Nathan Jones by punching Nathan in the groin.

Side of quads: located 5 inches above the knee can cause great pain. You can strike with roundhouse kick.

Center of quad: you can cause pain with a front kick or side-kick.

Knees: kicking someone's knee to the side can cause a tear that will disable any attacker. You can perform an outside to inwards roundhouse kick. Chen Zhen (Jet Li) finishes General Fujita with a knee strike in the "Fist of Legend" movie.

Ankle: there are pressure points on inside and outside of ankle that can be hit with leg sweep. Near the end of fight between Bruce Lee and Chuck Norris in "Way of the Dragon" movie, Bruce weakens Chuck with a leg sweep causing Chuck to fall.

Big toe: you can stomp on attacker's big toe if they are grabbing you from behind.

9 MOVE SELF DEFENSE COMBO

When faced with danger, causing the most damage to the threat in the least amount of time and energy allows you more time to escape and call the police. Practice this 9 move combination to buy you 30 seconds for each move landed which is 4.5 minutes that should allow you to escape on foot or car quickly. In a left forward fighting position stance: 1. left palm strike to the nose. 2. while attacker protects nose, right front kick to the groin. 3. while stepping down to front with right foot, right hammer fist with tremendous force to right side of neck. 4. quickly followed by left elbow with full body twist to right side of jaw. 5. while attacker is leaning away to their left, reload for strong left hook punch to right temple. 6. while attacker is protecting their head, right shuffle low side kick to their right knee. 7. while attacker grabs right knee, throw a left elbow to right jaw and right uppercut to chin combo. 8. while attacker holds face, left roundhouse liver kick to right ribcage. 9. while attacker grabs their right rib, finish with left spinning hook kick to the left temple. Done.

PART II

ATHLETIC (SUPERSTAR)

If you have everything under control, you're not moving fast enough

- Mario Andretti

CHAPTER 10

GLOBAL OBESITY

We are the champions, my friends. And we'll keep on fighting til the end...No time for losers 'cause we are the champions of the world.

- Queen in song "We Are The Champions"

OLYMPIC MOTIVATION

Being proactive is an ability possessed by the motivated as most people are reactive, taking action after a disaster such as an obesity or diabetes diagnosis. Per the United States Federal Government, only 20% of Americans get enough exercise and childhood obesity has prompted the United States to encourage young children to exercise to prevent poor health later in life.

Earth has a serious global health issue. Per the World Health Organization, over 400 million people worldwide have diabetes and 2.1 billion people are overweight. 15% of diabetics experience nerve damage in foot caused by elevated glucose levels leading to foot ulcers. More dangerous is 25% of people with foot ulcers undergo lower extremity amputation (LEA) where they have to cut their foot off - which has a lifetime cost of $500,000 in medical expenses. There are currently 2 million people living in the United States with limb loss. At America's current rate, 9 out of 10 Americans will be overweight by 2030. Fortunately over 90% of diabetics are type 2 who can improve their health thru nutrition and exercise. JustHuynh Fitness' mission is to help over 2 billion overweight people improve fitness to thrive in life.

In America, the CDC (Centers for Disease Control and Prevention) calls physical activity the "wonder drug." The President's Council is charged with increasing awareness about exercise which will help prevent heart conditions, Type II diabetes, arthritis, depression, dementia, anxiety, certain types of cancer and other chronic diseases. Maintaining an active lifestyle leads to societal benefits as well where active children perform better in school and have fewer social issues related to bullying, teen pregnancy and violence. Adults who are active have lower rates of absenteeism and are more productive in the workplace.

Sports can help casual couch potato fans turn into healthy exercisers. Every four years, the Summer Olympics and World Cup are sensational events where fans pack their cities cheering on their favorite athletes from their countries. The individual sport that brings countries together annually 4 times a year is tennis with superstars Serena Williams, Roger Federer, Maria Sharapova, and Rafael Nadal dominating the headlines.

Football, known as soccer in the United States, is a huge event in the summer where communities around the world band together to cheer on the 11 men representing their respective countries to win the elusive World Cup Champion title. As a kid, everyone dreams of one day winning the World Cup for their country. The excitement even for overweight people is evident in 2018 when Mexico defeated Germany in the Group Stage. When the winning goal was scored by Mexico, the entire nation jumped up and down creating a powerful force thought as an Earthquake. That should inspire you to exercise and share joys - hopefully not Earth shaking.

Then there is the Summer Olympics typically dominated by the United States, China, and Russia. During the Rio 2016 Olympic Games, there were 28 different sports including the popular track & field, swimming, and basketball. When victory comes down to the last point or hundredths of a second, that gets people's adrenaline going.

Sadly once these International Competitions finish, most people go back to their normal sedentary couch potato life. Starting today, instead of being a casual fan on the sidelines, motivate yourself to stay healthy so you can be a "World Champion" in life personally and professionally. The United States Federal Government encourages preschoolers ages 3 through 5 to be active at least 3 hours throughout the day. Children ages 6 thru 17 should exercise at least 1 hour a day with 3 of those days including muscle and bone strengthening activities like climbing on playground equipment or playing sports. Adult over age 18 should exercise at least 5 hour a week with 2 days consisting of muscle-strengthening exercise like push-ups or weight lifting.

AMERICAN SPORTS CALENDAR

Sports playoffs, the Summer Olympics, and the World Cup motivate fans to get off the sidelines and focus on their own health. Mark down these events to draw motivation throughout the year. In January (NFL football playoffs), March (college basketball "March Madness" tournament), May (NHL hockey playoffs), June (NBA basketball playoffs), July (FIFA soccer World Cup), August (Summer Olympics), September (Tennis U.S. Open),

October (MLB baseball world series), and December (college football "bowl" games).

LEADERSHIP ZERO TO HERO MOTIVATION

Sports and fitness builds character. By being a part of a team, you have the opportunity to achieve greatness together and be recognized by your peers as a leader in guiding the team to win. By "leading by example" on the field, you will have the support of your peers because "walk the talk." Acquiring this leadership experience as a great individual or team sports player translates into business. In business, leaders are generally the people who receive positive feedback from their employees, peer leaders, and bosses. Leaders are typically the person you'll notice in an office where employees seek advice for sales, customer satisfaction, partner respect, and employee approval.

After winning multiple Super Bowls with the New England Patriots, Tom Brady paid it forward by delivering an inspiring speech to his former college - University of Michigan. Tom said he used to be a student just like them who grew up into the leader he is today saying "I didn't have an easy experience. I didn't come in as a top rated recruit. I didn't come in with the opportunity to play right away. I had to earn it. And you know what the greatest honor I've ever received as a player is? In my 4th year and my 5th year, I was named team captain. That to this day is the single greatest achievement I've ever had as a football player. Because the men in this room chose me to lead their team. These were the guys that knew that I liked to work, that knew I loved football, that knew I loved to play...all those lessons I learned in college is what I still bring to practice today. After 14 years, I love the game more than I have ever loved it. But where did I learn the love for the game? Where did I learn to practice? Where did I learn to compete? It was sitting in the same chairs that you guys are sitting in today."

CHAMPIONSHIP MOTIVATION - PATRIOTS

Many people go thru life saying "F*ck My Life" as they are stuck in jobs they don't like so aren't able to enjoy waking up in the morning everyday.

Negative attitudes can lead to a downward spiral of unhealthy habits such as drinking alcohol, smoking, eating fat foods, not exercising, being passed over by women or men for love, not getting the pay you deserve, and doing drugs. Being fit changes everything because you get to be a "champion for life." As Imi said in his "Krav Maga" book, "the fat rich guy with a young beautiful girlfriend by his side would die for the athletic healthy body of a poor circus gymnast" - realizing that being healthy has many benefits in life.

In football, old players or overlooked players who have never won a championship in their life, take lower pay for the chance of winning a Super Bowl for their first time with Tom Brady. These players know that your life changes when you become a "champion." In Super Bowl 51 in 2017, Tom Brady became the quarterback with the most Super Bowl titles in NFL history with 5 after rallying his team back from a 28-3 deficit to the Atlanta Falcons known as "the greatest Super Bowl of all-time." After winning their first championship, Tom Brady's teammates typically leave to sign million dollar contracts with other teams who want someone with championship experience to motivate the 53 men. For example backup quarterback Jimmy Garoppolo, who has 7 career NFL starts compared to Tom Brady's 9 Super Bowl appearances, became the highest paid quarterback by signing a 5-year $137.5 million contract with the San Francisco 49ers. In business, this is similar to companies who poach former Amazon and Facebook executives to get the inside scoop of how Jeff Bezos and Mark Zuckerberg run their "championship" companies.

JustHuynh Fitness' online training program and studio classes can help you become a champion in life as well.

Before Super Bowl 51, long-time Tom Brady and New England Patriots rival and hater Ray Lewis delivered a garage pre-game speech to motivate the Patriots in their quest for 5 Super Bowls. Reference this motivational speech if you ever feel tired of winning or want to have a championship DNA.

Ray Lewis said "People telling us that we're okay with losing. Champions never be OK with losing. 5 rings! 5 rings says everything for what we've built. What we've done. It's never about the wins and losses - it's about the opportunity to be a champion for the rest of your life! That's what the New England Patriots believe in. That's what our culture is. And guest what? It may be us against the world, but who cares?! Today is all that matters...4th quarter! Real champions find a way to win because of fundamentals. That's why we're so doggone good...regardless if you like us, you better respect us! Because if you don't! I promise you the scoreboard will. This is a chance to capture a legacy that's forever...Once you hold the Lombardi Trophy...You will know that the New England Patriots are probably the greatest team of all time...It's your time now Brady. It's your time leader. It's your time general. Lead us to the next place. You've done it for so long! Somebody's trying to come take your throne. You must make this personal! This has to be personal! Everybody's saying your okay because you've already won four. Look around this locker room and look in these men's eyes...and let them see why you were picked in the 6th round! Let them see what that passion feels like! Today, we're crowned as the champions of the world. Five! New England Patriots - Let's Go!"

MEASURING OBESITY - BMI

Humans are one of the most fascinating species in the world as our weight affects our self image. People understand that being healthy helps one feel and look good, but putting that knowledge to action is tough.

Fitless people, as portrayed in the movie "Wall-E," possess physical deficiencies that lead to an unfulfilling personal life and business career. Plato said "To succeed in life, perfection is achieved thru education and exercise." Having a fit body sharpens your mind to pursue your dreams.

So how do you know whether you're overweight or obese? The standard assessment for people older than 20 is called the Body Mass Index known as the BMI that is a measure of body fat based on your weight in relation to your height. Being overweight is defined as having a BMI greater than or equal to 25 and lower than 30, while obesity is defined as having a BMI equal to or greater than 30.

America is #1 globally in many categories such as having the most prestigious universities and disposable income, but is also #1 in the wrong categories such as having the worst life expectancy, infant mortality, and obesity rate in the world.

Global Obesity or "Globesity" as coined by the World Health Organization (WHO) is real with 9 out of 10 Americans expected to be overweight by 2030. Currently, ⅓ of the world or 2.1 billion adults are overweight.

When looking at obesity alone (BMI over 30), America is the fattest in the world with 35% of the population or 78 million obese adults. China follows at a distant second with 46 million obese and India third with 30 million obese adults.

The 2008 Disney Film "Wall E" depicted the future obese world with people hovering around in mobility scooters watching ads and sipping soft drinks all day. 10 years later in 2018, Hollywood is not too far off from reality with people streaming TV from their couch 4 hours a day as if watching TV was their part-time job, wasting their time in a virtual world playing Fortnite shooting game, or scrolling thru social media for depression.

Not caring for your waistline will kill your bottom line as evident with the United States spending $344 billion of healthcare budget on obesity in 2018 which is 20% of the total healthcare budget. Being overweight (BMI > 25) increases your susceptibility to health risks such as cardiovascular disease, cancer, diabetes, osteoarthritis, and chronic kidney disease. It's worth knowing that 70% of deaths are lifestyle related and preventable, but people still fail to be proactive with their fitness resulting in 17.5 million people dying annually from cardiovascular disease - the equivalent of four jumbo jets or 2,000 people crashing every hour, every single day, every year.

BELLY BOOTY BREAST HEALTH RISKS

In general, women have greater absolute body fat percentages than men. Typically, women carry more fat around the legs, hip, buttocks, chest, and upper arms. Here are other common body parts where you may find fat.

Thunder thighs are something you should be proud of. A study by the British Medical Journal "Large Thighs Protect Against Heart Disease and Early Death" found that men and women whose thighs are less than 60 centimeters (23.6 inches) in circumference have a higher risk of premature death and heart disease. As such doctors recommend patients not to forget leg day to increase their thigh size.

A big booty is fine according to an Oxford University study suggesting that a big booty helps protect you from diabetes and heart disease. The idea is that lower-body fat in your thighs, hips, and buttocks traps fatty acids from the foods you eat so they don't float through your bloodstream and get deposited in organs to harm you.

Magazines tend to depict having big breasts as attractive but it's actually unhealthy per a Harvard University and University of Toronto joint study of more than 92,000 women showing that women with big breasts were at greater risk of type 2 diabetes. Women who have a D cup at age 20 were three times more likely to develop diabetes as they aged.

If you think that going thru belly surgery or a fad diet is all you need for a slim body without any exercise, think again. Putting time in the weight room helps build the necessary muscles that burn calories faster than other tissues. Muscle cells are also more responsive to insulin - lowering blood sugar levels without requiring the high insulin levels that are associated with high cardiovascular risk.

There are two kinds of fat in this world. One is subcutaneous - the layer of fat cells under your skin that your body uses to store fuel. Subcutaneous fat is the squishy fat just under the surface of your skin that jiggles when you walk and isn't considered hazardous. The other type of fat is dangerous called visceral (belly) fat which are fat cells that accumulate inside the body in and around your organs. Visceral fat secretes greater levels of adipokines – chemicals that trigger inflammation – and releases more fatty acids into the bloodstream that can put you at risk of heart disease, type 2 diabetes, high blood pressure, cancer, and dementia.

When you buy life insurance or get your annual medical check, a health professional can tell if you possess a dangerous amount of belly fat by measuring your waist. If your waist measures 35 or more inches for women or 40 or more inches for men, you possess a dangerous amount of belly fat.

What makes belly (visceral) fat so harmful? Your liver can borrow the visceral fat to turn it into cholesterol that can slip into your bloodstream and start collecting along your arteries. Increased cholesterol causes the arteries to harden that can lead to a heart attack or stroke. Belly fat also causes the body to become insulin-resistant, raises your glucose levels, and decreases your muscle mass.

Until midlife, men usually have a greater percentage of visceral fat than women, but the pattern reverses as women pass through menopause. Few females escape the midlife waistline expansion as body fat redistributes and visceral fat pushes out our bellies. Aging plays a role where you lose muscle if you don't exercise. Loss of muscle mass decreases the rate at which your body uses calories - making it challenging to maintain a healthy weight.

The Million Women Study conducted in Britain demonstrated a direct link between the development of coronary heart disease and an increase in waist circumference over a 20-year period where every additional two inches in the women's waist size raised their heart disease risk by 10 percent.

A study of 6,583 members of Kaiser Permanente of Northern California who were followed for an average of 36 years found that those with the greatest amount of abdominal obesity in midlife were three times likely to develop dementia than those with the least abdominal fat in thirty years.

KILLING BELLYFAT

Exercise is the all-natural remedy to kill bellyfat over fad diets or belly surgery. Dr. Ronald Kahn (the George Richards Minot Professor of Medicine at Harvard Medical School) says he doesn't talk with patients about going on a diet but more about creating a long-term lifestyle program that includes physical activity and sustainable dietary changes. Weight that comes off slowly tends to stay off whereas rapid weight loss triggers your body to slow its metabolism, setting the stage for the weight to be regained quickly otherwise known as a "yo-yo dieter."

Dr. Francisco Lopez-Jimenez, of the Mayo Clinic in Minnesota, says 30 minutes of exercise six days a week is sufficient to keep belly fat off. As for eating, you should have fruits, vegetables and whole grains with lean sources of protein such as fish and low-fat dairy products. You should avoid foods with added sugar, processed carbohydrates, and empty calories from alcohol.

Rest and low stress also help with reducing belly fat. People who regularly get 6-7 hours of sleep each night tend to have lower measures of visceral fat.

PLASTIC SURGERY

People often wasted days, weeks, months, and years in building up belly fat. For some reason, people have the notion that one day of exercise can eliminate yearsworths of bad habits. As such, many Americans don't like what they see in the mirror and keep plastic surgeons busy fueling the $16 billion cosmetic surgery industry with 17.5 million cosmetic and minimally-invasive procedures performed in 2017 for Americans according to statistics from the American Society of Plastic Surgeons (ASPS). Plastic surgery isn't all women as men accounted for 13.8% of cosmetic procedures - favoring eyelid and breast reduction (man boobs) surgeries.

Fat grafting is most popular where plastic surgeons harvest a patient's unwanted fat from their abdomen using liposuction and then injecting that unwanted fat to lift other areas of the body such as the face, butt, and even the breast said ASPS President Debra Johnson.

In 2017, there were 235,237 liposuction surgeries performed in U.S. at average cost if $3,200 and 127,633 Tummy Tuck procedures were performed at average cost of $5,798.

Inspired by Instagram Stars Kim Kardashian for her breasts and butt and Dwayne Johnson for his arms, both men and women put themselves under the knife in other body parts as well.

For breasts per Navin Singh, a plastic surgeon with offices in McLean and Chevy Chase, women want to address the saggy breast with "teardrop" shaping as opposed to stuffing the breast with implants. Thru exercise, you can achieve your desired breast size thru push-ups, pull-ups, seated cable rows, and incline bench presses.

As for the butt, the "Brazilian Butt Lift (BBL)" is favored where a surgeon removes unwanted fat from elsewhere in the body (commonly the hips, thighs, or belly) and uses that fat to smooth, shape, and elevate the butt. A BBL costs on average $9,000 - with swelling plus four to six weeks of wearing a compression garment. You can enhance your butt naturally thru exercise by performing squats and lunges.

If you want to get rid of saggy arms to build muscular biceps like Dwayne Johnson, a brachioplasty can reshape your saggy upper arms for average cost of $6,500. Thru exercise, back to back moves between biceps and triceps such as bicep concentration curls and overhead tricep arm extensions can help you get muscular arms.

One of our female clients wanted to address her droopy breasts, saggy arms, and jiggly butt. By committing to 3 days of cardio and 3 days of strength training a week with JustHuynh Fitness' signature martial arts and power athletics, she saw results as quickly as 1 month. The power of commitment can go a long way as long as you're willing to enjoy the journey in achieving your desired physical results without having to resort to plastic surgery as the first option to eliminate fat.

CHAPTER 11

FITNESS METRICS

Eating healthy food, watching your weight, and exercise should be a lifetime habit - best begun when you are as young as possible

- Clint Eastwood

HEALTH WARNINGS

If you're still just checking the box unsatisfied in life with your 9-5 job or going thru stress, here are acronym indicators inspired by wolves to signal when "enough is enough" to not let life push you around anymore - signalling it is time to prioritize fitness.

Miserable people often resort to fat foods (BMI), alcohol (BAC), and drugs (FSL) to escape life's harsh reality. For wolf analogy featured in films, you could have an obese BMI (Body Mass Index) greater than 30 like Chubby in "Teen Wolf" movie, a high BAC (Blood Alcohol Content) making it dangerous to drive and interact socially like the guys in the "Hangover" movie series, or experience death from too much drugs that put you in FSL (fundamental state of leadership) likes the "Wolf of Wall Street" film featuring Leonardo Dicaprio, Jonah Hill, and Matthew McConaughey.

MENTAL FITNESS

To get your life back together it's important to work on improving your mental fitness. Here are mental metrics that you should prioritize.
- Love: you have a significant other to share your life with
- Intelligence: read a book a month to learn new things and work your brain.
- Alcohol: no alcohol in your life
- Drugs: no drugs in your life
- Smoking: no smoking in your life
- Bullying: don't attack anyone verbally online or physically offline
- TV: watch to relax but don't approach the dangerous average of 4

hours a day - treating watching TV like its a part-time job
- Social Media: use just for connecting with friends not a time waster
- Video Games: eliminate games and start interacting with people

PHYSICAL METRICS

Here are physical metrics to prioritize
- BMI: between 18.5 and 24.9
- Army Fitness Test: score greater than 70 points in all events
- Age Guess: strangers guess that you look 10 years younger than your actual age. That's a compliment to the benefits of exercise
- Insurance: low premium spend as you don't need to visit the hospital
- Pills: eliminate prescription pills especially for weight loss or Type 2 diabetes where your body is healthy thru exercise
- Dining Out: limit to healthy meals. Call the restaurant ahead of time for health options to order
- Daily Calories Consumed: commit to 1,500 to 1,800 calories a day with essential macronutrients obtained thru food, supplements, and vitamin pills
- Maximum Heart Rate: exercise at 65% maximum heart rate for 12 minutes six times per week
- Weekly Fitness: perform cardio 3 times per week and resistance training 3 times per week

ATHLETIC DEVELOPMENT - VO2 MAX

There are 3 measurements to focus on for improving your speed (300 meter sprint), endurance (Vo2 Max), and power (Kicking Power).

For your 300 meter time, try to get at least 1 point on the FBI Personal Fitness Test standards for males (faster than 52.4 seconds) and females (faster than 54.9 seconds). Getting at least 1 point ensures that you have a healthy heart.

The VO2 max is globally used as an indicator of health. In 2016, the American Heart Association published a scientific statement recommending that cardiorespiratory fitness (CRF), quantifiable as VO2 max, be regularly assessed as a clinical vital sign. People with low fitness levels are susceptible to cardiovascular disease.

You can improve your VO2 thru the Cooper test which involves running as far as you can in 12 minutes. This is a conditioning test used by world cup soccer teams, American NFL players, and American college basketball players. On a 400 meter track, men able to run at least six laps (2,400 meters) and women able to run at least five lap (2,000 meters) have great endurance and are likely to see lower healthcare costs and reduced chances of heart disease.

In physics, Newton's law of motion states that force equals mass times acceleration. At JustHuynh Fitness, our boxing and kickboxing program helps people build confidence and self defense skills while burning calories and gaining muscle efficiently. The goal is for anyone to execute a back-leg mid-body roundhouse kick with 1,000 pounds of devastating force power. To reach this goal, practice kicking without and with the bag, strengthen your shins, sprint, strengthen your core, and perform lower body leg exercises.

HEART RATE MONITORS TO BURN FAT

Your heart, measured by the amount of times it beats per minute, is a muscle that becomes stronger as you exercise more. The harder you exercise your muscles, more oxygen is required which is supplied to your muscles from your lungs via the bloodstream. As such, your heart pumps faster during a workout to deliver the additional oxygen needed by your muscles.

Before using a heart rate monitor, it's important for you to understand the 4 different types of heart rates to set realistic training goals.

Resting Heart Rate: Your resting heart rate (RHR) is your heart's beats per minute when you're relaxed. Although heart rates vary between individuals, the average RHR for a man is between 60 to 80 beats per minute and 70 to 90 beats per minute for a woman. A healthy adult can have an RHR in the low 60's while an unhealthy RHR can be as high as 100.

Maximum Heart Rate: Your maximum heart rate (MHR) is the peak amount of beats that your heart can reach during a workout. To calculate your maximum heart rate, subtract your age from the number 220. If you're 30, your MHR would be 190. Note that this formula is not an exact science.

Training Heart Rate: Your training heart rate (THR) is the rate that you should maintain during aerobic workouts in an effort to improve fitness. To enhance fitness, you can train from 55 to 85 percent of your maximum heart rate for 20-30 minutes each workout. If you're 30 years old with a MHR of 190, your THR range would be 104.5 to 161.5. Training in this THR range will trigger your body to burn fat.

To tap into your body's "after-burn" effect of burning upwards of 200 additional calories for 36 hours after your workout and to enhance athletic performance, exercise in THR above 85% of your MHR for 12 minutes of your workout. High-intensity interval training (HIIT) workouts thru martial arts, boot-camps, and speed athletics can help you train above 85% of your MHR.

Recovery Heart Rate: Your recovering heart rate is the rate that you should bring your heart down to after a workout. A good number to go by is 20 beats within your pre-workout resting heart rate.

How Heart Rate Monitors Work: The most effective monitors measure your heart rate with a transmitter that is placed over the heart and held in place by an adjustable strap that wraps around your chest. Individuals need to listen to their heart and train at the right intensity. Heart rate monitors also provide other useful fitness insights such as calorie burn stats.

PHYSICAL FITNESS TEST - FBI & ARMY

Performing Physical Fitness Tests every couple months helps you assess improvements in your physical and mental fitness. At JustHuynh Fitness, we recommend our clients undergo the FBI Physical Fitness Test or the Army Combat Readiness Test every 2 months. Physical fitness tests ensure that clients are benefiting from our target heart rate training and martial arts programming.

STATE OF THE UNITED STATES MILITARY

With the 3rd largest Army in the World - behind China and India, the United States' 1.4 million soldiers must be physically and mentally tough to fight and win in high intensity conflict.

In 2018, the United States Army had a target of 76,500 recruits, but missed its recruiting target for the first time since 2005 - falling short by 6,500 soldiers. Despite high tech military challenges from China and Russia, the Pentagon has admitted to a fast-growing national security threat of obesity where 71% of Americans age 17-24 are overweight. General Mark Milley stated that the United States doesn't want young men and women getting killed in action because they were too fat to fight.

With $1.5 billion spent annually on obese unfit soldiers, Defense Secretary James Mattis has enacted a "deploy-or-be-removed" policy where troops who are non-deployable for more than 12 months will be processed for administrative separation. At one point, 15% or about 150,000 soldiers were categorized as non-deployable.

Fitness success can be achieved regardless of age or gender as the enemy shows no remorse for your physical or mental deficiencies. In Hollywood classic "Full Metal Jacket," Private Pyle's training is inspiring for any soldier looking to pass the Army's fitness expectations.

With many soldiers injured due to poor fitness, the United States studied foreign militaries who have successful physical fitness tests such as the Australian Army who saw a 30% reduction in injuries. Israel is another good example as it is one of the few countries in the world with mandatory military service for women. If you search YouTube, you'll see talk show host Conan O'Brien appreciating the might of the Israeli Women Soldiers.

With that, U.S. Military Training lead scientist Whitfield East was asked to revise the outdated 1980 Army Physical Fitness Test by assessing five of the hardest warrior tasks like evacuating casualties from a vehicle, moving under and around obstacles, and hand-to-hand combat. Reverse-engineering these combat specific tasks using regression analysis led to five domains of physical fitness: muscular endurance, cardiovascular endurance, muscular strength, explosive strength, and agility.

STATE OF THE CHINESE MILITARY

A rising number of Chinese people are failing military fitness tests because they are too fat, eat poorly and masturbate too much - according to a report published in state-run military newspaper "the People's Liberation Army Daily." Authorities believe the constant use of smartphones caused 46 per cent of candidates to fail the vision test.

STATE OF THE RUSSIAN MILITARY

In 2016, Russia ranked third in the world for military spending at $69.2 billion - behind the United States' $611 billion and China's $215 billion; and ahead of Saudi Arabia's $63.7 billion and India's $55.9 billion.

Concerned for his country in 2013, Judoka Vladimir Putin called for the revival of the 1931 Soviet-era physical evaluation program that required all schoolchildren to pass fitness tests called the GTO which is a Russian acronym for "Ready for Labor and Defense" where children learn "to stand up for themselves, their family and their Fatherland." After the Soviet collapse in 1991, schools were on their own in improving their student's health. In response, Russia's Sports Minister Vitaly Mutko planned to introduce physical training standards nationwide by 2016. One year ahead of time in 2015,

Vladimir Putin signed GTO into law to standardize physical development in areas such as running, swimming, biking, shooting and trekking skills. To make training accessible, Russia spent $18 million on training centers.

In 2018, the Russian military released photos of the Russian special task force participating in a 5-mile cross country race (soldiers go thru chest-high swamps, carry thick and heavy logs with other soldiers, prove strength by carrying a comrade on their shoulders while walking thru a hip-high section of water, and dodge bullets from small firearms), weapon skills showcase, and 12 minutes-of-hell boxing matches (four 3-minute rounds against different maroon berets) while being verbally abused to earn their maroon beret in online articles titled "Russian soldiers batter each other in bloody boxing bouts."

U.S. ARMY COMBAT READINESS TEST

For the first time since 1980, in 2018 the United States revised the Army Combat Readiness Test that is gender and age neutral as war doesn't distinguish between gender and age. Military Training Command Sergeant Edward Mitchell says "You can be 20 years old on the battlefield or you can be 50 and you're going to have to accomplish the same mission. This test helps you execute your warrior tasks and battle drills, no matter who you are."

The 1980 Army Physical Test only accounted for 40% of warrior tasks whereas the 2018 Army Combat Readiness accounts for 80% of warrior tasks. The United States Army's goal is for the new test to reduce injury rates especially musculoskeletal which accounts for billions of dollars every year in terms of health care costs for active duty and veteran soldiers. Secretary of the Army Mark T. Esper says "If you can't pass the Army Combat Fitness Test, then there's probably not a spot for you in the Army. At the end of the day, the United States needs Soldiers who are deployable, lethal, and ready."

The 2018 Army Combat Readiness test is a 6 event exam to be completed in 50 minutes. The 6 events consist of a 3-rep hexbar deadlift, a 10lb backward toss, release pushups, a 250 meter Sprint/Drag/Carry, hanging leg tucks, and 2 mile run. You can find scoring guidelines online.

Taking the fitness test for the first time, my total score would be 240 lb deadlift (82pts), 10lb backward toss 10.1 meter (81pts), 50 hand release pushups (90pts), 1:50 Sprint/Drag/Carry (89pts), 20 leg tucks (100pts), and 13:44 2 mile run (95pts) for total of 537 points or 89.5% total points.

In regards to my physical fitness test experience, I've passed the FBI Physical Fitness in 2016, performed the Cooper Fitness test with the Boston

Police, and completed the Super Soldier joint-study with Natick Soldier Research and Tuft University. With a background in martial arts and sprinting, JustHuynh Fitness can help you pass the Army Combat Readiness Test for military service or physical fitness goals thru our studio and online programs.

SPORTS COMPETITIONS

After college, many adults lose the convenience of organized activities at their university to play pick-up soccer, basketball, football, or other sports they enjoy. By focusing on improving your 300 meter time, VO2 max, and kicking power, you can perform well and even win competitions ranging from a pickup soccer game, a 5,000 meter run, individual sports like tennis or golf, and obstacle course races.

For optimal performance, every day that you step onto the track, fighting ring, sports arena, or business office, you should think about what your opponent is doing. In your mind, outwork and outsmart your opponent. Thru JustHuynh Fitness, your opponents will break down in the 4th quarter due to their poor conditioning so you speed past them for victory.

CHAPTER 12

KILLING OBESITY 3 TIMES

We must all suffer from one of two pains: the pain of discipline or the pain of regret. The difference is discipline weighs ounces while regret weighs tons

- Jim Rohn

OBESITY PHASES IN LIFE

Per the World Health Organization (WHO), over 400 million people worldwide have diabetes of which 30 million are from the United States. You, your family, and friends who cast aside health put yourself at risk of obesity, diabetes, cancer, and even death. Fortunately over 90% of diabetics are type 2 who can improve their health thru nutrition and exercise.

Having personally overcome obesity 3 times in life: childhood (Age 10), college Freshman 15 (Age 18), and corporate (Age 22) from staying in hotels and eating out 200 nights a year for 4 consecutive years, I got the wakeup call during my annual health physical weighing in at 160 pounds for a 5'2"guy - which is obese (29.3 BMI) on an Asian BMI scale.

CHILDHOOD OBESITY

Children Age 2 to Teenagers Age 19 can determine if they are overweight or obese using the Center of Disease Control and Prevention (CDC) BMI calculator.

Per the Organization of Economic Cooperation and Development (OECD), 1 in 6 children are overweight. Obese children are more likely to develop a variety of health problems when they become adults including cardiovascular disease, insulin resistance (a sign of prediabetes), musculoskeletal disorders (especially osteoarthritis), some cancers (endometrial, breast and colon), and disability.

Social influences at home and school are leading forces of child obesity. At home, children who are raised by obese parents have an 80% chance of being obese when they become adults. That is a staggering statistic. Parents must lead by example by serving nutritious meals and storing healthy foods at home. A house full of junk food and daily orders of fast food is a fast track to obesity.

Children grow up idolizing athletes and hollywood stars seen on television. Parents must do their best to curb television viewership as food and beverage companies spend billions of marketing dollars targeting kids to influence their food choices.

New York University conducted research on sports sponsorships discovering that major sports leagues like the NFL and NBA have millions of young viewers (about 412 million under the age of 17 per year). Unfortunately, the vast majority of the snacks and drinks featured through these sponsorships are unhealthy. Kids see these pro athletes at the pinnacle of physical fitness — then the television cuts to a commercial for chips and sugary drinks which leading kids to think these products are healthier than they are when 76% of food and beverage ads shown are unhealthy such as Snickers bars, Doritos chips, and Frosted Flake cereals. When kids see a given food branded with a superhero or a sports hero, they eat more of it.

As parents, you can take charge in your community similar to the World Health Organization who suggest strict regulations on food ads targeted at kids. Bans on advertising of foods and beverages on TV and radio during hours when children are the main audience have been put in place in Chile, Iceland, Ireland, and Mexico. Other bans apply in schools (e.g. Chile, Poland, Spain and Turkey), in public transport (e.g. Australia) and other public places (e.g. Norway). In America, cities such as Phoenix applied to earn grants nationally to fight obesity in their communities.

Being obese as children in school is tough as children face low odds of enjoying benefits of normal weight, experience social discrimination for being overweight by their classmates, and likely to obtain medical problems.

Food education should be a part of the curriculum where students can visit local farms, learn about healthy eating and cooking.

For exercise, John Ratey's book "Spark" covered a wonderful success story from Naperville, IL in 1999 where all middle schools implemented a gym class for 19,000 students transforming them into the fittest middle-schoolers in the nation as only 3% of Naperville was overweight vs the 30% national average. Best of all was the benefits of the benefits to the mind with improved intelligence where Naperville's 8th graders took the TIMSS

(Trends in International Mathematics and Science Study) test against powerhouses of China, Japan, and Singapore - beating them out for 1st in Science and 6th in Math worldwide.

Childhood obesity is personal as I was obese at Age 10 with little exercise and bad nutrition. Seeing that, my father enrolled me in karate for 3 years and signed us up for the track team as it's the only sport that doesn't make cuts! I'm forever grateful for my father's encouragement to exercise as I became healthier and improved academically finishing top 10 in high school, attended an elite liberal arts college in Maine, and graduated with honors from MBA business school. Without exercise, I would not be where I am today to pay it forward with a personal mission to help 2 billion overweight people become healthier.

For students, the call to action is to exercise for 60 minutes 3 times a week, eat healthily, and be careful of the unhealthy advertisements seen on television by superheros and athletes you love.

Fitness can be a family sport or community-driven thru your school or sports team. If your family is ready to rid yourself of obesity, reach out to our JustHuynh Fitness for online and studio group fitness programs.

COLLEGE OBESITY

In 2017, there were 20.4 million college students in America who will or have experienced the "Freshman 15" which is the human experience of putting on 15 pounds of body weight during their first year in college. For students, this is their first time living away from their parents or guardian without home-made food. On college campuses, students encounter several challenges relating to nutrition, exercise, and mental health.

For nutrition, most students are on a buffet-style campus meal-plan where students can have seconds and more - leading to more calories than they should be eating. When eating on campus, students must stay disciplined with portion size and not go get seconds.

Outside of the dining hall, students garf down pizza, soda, and beer at student club meetings and parties. This is an easy way to put on unhealthy weight. When going to a meeting or party, bring a healthy snack or a nutritious cold meal with you to eat when you feel hungry. It's also important to replace sleepless benders with solid sleep.

With over 7 billion people, college students typically feel stuck in a "campus bubble" secluded from the "outside world" where they must follow the crowd or risk being criticized by their friends. Don't feel pressured to drink alcohol at college parties - convince others it is cool to be fit, healthy, and smart by drinking water.

Some of the most successful people are college dropouts: Steve Jobs, Bill Gates, Mark Zuckerberg. They weren't concerned with peer pressure as they knew their purpose and plan outside of the college bubble.

Packing on the weight from junk food and beer makes exercise a tough habit to make. College students have additional no-time excuses ranging from class, homework, club activities, career search, hangovers, social media, online shopping, "Netflix and Chilling," and partying. Everyone has the same 24 hours in a day. If a busy person like President Barack Obama managed to exercise, you can too.

If you attend a college where college athletes are the "Big Man or Big Woman on Campus," you probably cheer on the football and basketball teams during big games, but don't be afraid of their presence if you work out in the gym. The majority of college athletes don't make it professionally often just reflecting on their glory days while working a subpar job because they didn't focus on their career plans while in college. Hollywood captured this with Dwayne Johnson and Kevin Hart in the movie "Central Intelligence." Remember to have a mindset beyond the campus bubble to get in your exercise so you can go pursue your dreams after finishing college.

I too went thru the college freshman 15 at Bowdoin College - consistently ranked the top dining hall in the United States. My exercise slipped from high school as I used all those time excuses mentioned earlier such as studying and partying. To overcome this, I started controlling portion size every meal and ate healthily when out socially. For exercise, learning how to structure a weight lifting program from my roommate helped me realize the benefits of lifting to boost metabolism and physique. Training with partners helped for social accountability and motivation. Go find your partner! Mental health is a huge issue where students can go thru depression or commit suicide for low grades or not succeeding with their Tinder-swiping dating life on campus.

At college, what other students think of you may seem like the most important thing in the world, but when you ask adults and your parents what they got wrong at that age, nearly all say they cared too much what other kids thought of them. Just ask anyone who's 5 years out of college if any of those peer pressure moments back then mattered now.

If you're someone who's packed on the college freshman 15 or want to avoid going thru it, start finding a friend who's willing to be disciplined with nutrition and exercise so you can enjoy the rest of your college experience to dominate after college with a great body and smarter mind.

If you, your friends, and college community are ready to take your college health to the next level, reach out to JustHuynh Fitness for online and studio group fitness programs. Feel free to invite your professors and school administrators too!

ADULT OBESITY

Only 23% of United States Adults get enough exercise per the CDC. Life is short where any second may be your last due to freak accident, mother nature, psychos, or self inflicted.

Worldwide, guess how many people are overweight vs starving? There are 600 million undernourished vs 2 billion overweight people.

Successful people prioritize fitness. Reducing your waistline will help increase your financial bottom line.

At work, workplace wellness programs have two main goals: improve employees' health and lower their employers' health-care costs. Turns out workplace wellness programs are not very good at either as studied by the National Bureau of Economic Research. The only employees taking advantage of financial incentives are people who are already healthy.

The US Department of Health and Human Services recommends that people between the ages of 18 and 64 exercise for at least 150 minutes each week spread over 3 days a week.

Successful companies generally have a dedicated leadership that is committed to wellness programs. Tim Cook of Apple works out at 5AM, Michelle Obama inspires children and adults thru her Let's Move initiative, and Jeff Bezos of Amazon - the richest person in the world now sports a fit physique to motivate his employees as they become the most dominant company in the world.

With the rise of jobs where people sit all day combined with addiction to phones after work, society is now lazy. Adult obesity is personal as I became obese for the 3rd time at age 22 from the brutal life on the road 200 nights a year. Healthwise, the 4 years of consulting travel were the worst as the hotel gyms had limited fitness equipment and nutrition consisted of drinking and eating huge meals everyday.

When back home from travels, I fell in the trap of most people checking the 9AM-5PM box during the weekdays to live for the weekends of heavy drinking on Friday and Saturday - using Sunday as recovery day to repeat the process again each week. It's a weekly vicious cycle that can kill you. In a rut personally and professionally, prioritizing nutrition and exercise helped me kill obesity for good. Within a year, I lowered my weight to 140 pounds for a 25.6 BMI which doctors approve as this BMI measure overestimates body fat for muscular and physically fit people - particular of Asian genetics.

With commitment to disciplined nutrition and exercise, I've been able to maintain this BMI level and health ever since - unlike those who gain all their lost weight back after participating in a fad diet program called yo-yo dieting. This happens time and time again as fad diets (cutting calories under 1,000 a day) don't work because it's temporary and not a permanent healthy lifestyle change. Life can be enjoyed without drinking. Today instead of Vodka, my favorite drink is water on the rocks.

As adults, it's in your company's best interest to invest in employee health to reduce healthcare costs while reaping the benefits that healthier employees boost the company's bottomline.

Many companies along with health insurance companies give employees money for tracking their steps with a pedometer. Unfortunately, employees cheat by tying their watch on a drone and flying it around to meet the steps goal. Companies also foster internal competition with month-long weight loss contests during New Year Resolution and the Summer. With money and bragging rights on the line, people go to extremes where employees gained 30 pounds by eating McDonalds so they could lose those 30 pounds to win the contest money.

Many companies and commercial real estate developers have on-site gyms as they know a healthy workforce reduces healthcare costs and improves productivity. However, the majority of gym equipment collects dust serving as amenity bragging rights against other companies for recruiting, but employees never use it. The first reason most people don't use the gym is due to laziness and another common reason people don't use onsite gyms is due to social stigma that you're showing off in front of lazy people.

To end all this laziness, JustHuynh Fitness provides online and studio group fitness programs. With nutrition as 70% and exercise as 30% of the battle, JustHuynh Fitness helps clients understand their causes for overeating and desire for unhealthy foods. Our goal is for you to break your bad habits and form healthy habits for life thru JustHuynh Fitness' brand of martial arts and power athletics.

CHAPTER 13

NATIONS FIGHT FAT

Even more people today have the means to live, but no meaning to live for

- Vicktor Frankl

FINLAND FAT TO FIT

In the 1970s, Finland was one of the world's unhealthiest nations. Diet was poor, people were inactive, and heart disease was at record levels. Everybody was smoking and eating lots of fat. Finnish men said vegetables were for rabbits so people simply did not eat vegetables instead resorted to butter on bread, whole fat milk, and fatty meat.

Amazingly, Finland halted the downward spiral towards terminal couch potatoism with community-based intervention. Instead of a mass campaign telling people what NOT to do, officials blitzed the population with positive incentives. Villages held "quit and win" competitions for smokers, where those who didn't smoke for a month won prizes. Entire towns competed against each other in cholesterol-cutting showdowns.

To succeed, local competitions were combined with sweeping nationwide legislation where all forms of tobacco advertising were banned. Farmers were forced to produce low-fat milk.

On exercise front, Finland built clean swimming pools, ball parks, and maintained snow parks to insert exercise into people's daily routines.

Based on your local and national circumstances, Finland is a great example of how local communities and national legislation can transform previously unhealthy populations into fit people.

JAPAN PREDIABETES EMPLOYER MANDATE

In 2008, Japan passed the "Metabo Law" designed to combat "metabolic syndrome," which is known to Americans as "pre-diabetes." The "Metabo Law" requires overweight individuals or individuals who show signs

---

of obesity or diabetes to take nutrition weight loss classes. If people fail to attend the classes, the companies including local governments who employ them must pay fines to the federal government. Furthermore, companies with more than a certain percentage of overweight employees are fined directly. If you travel to Japan which I did in 2018, you'll see first hand that most Japanese are fit which has resulted in the country having one of the longest human lifespans in the world.

Coupled with the fact that people on average waste 2 hours a day at work and waste 6 hours of their time each day, employers can gamify exercise similar to people walking outside to catch pokemon on "Pokemon Go" or employees feeling excited to answer trivia questions everyday with their co-workers on the game "HQ Trivia."

MEXICAN SUGAR TAX & SQUAT PASSES

In 2013, Mexico surpassed the United States as one of the fattest nations on the planet with 32.8% of the population obese. In response, its government announced a hefty tax on sugary drinks.

Inspired from Russia giving out free subway transportation tickets at the Sochi Winter Olympic Games for anyone who did 30 squats, Mexico installed 30 motion-sensitive machines at subway stations that dispenses a free subway ticket to anyone who completes 10 squats. Quick and easy.

CHINA PUBLIC GYMS

China's State Council approved the 2016-2020 National Fitness Plan as China is the 2nd most obese nation in the world with 57 million obese adults. The National Fitness Program introduces a "new national consciousness of health and fitness" by encouraging citizens of all ages to incorporate physical exercise into their lives. The "sports facility network" places a fitness or sports center within one mile of every resident.

RUSSIAN READY FOR LABOR AND DEFENSE

In 2014, President Vladimir Putin announced that a Stalinist fitness program from the 1930s called "Ready for Labor and Defense (GTO)" will be revived and funded by leftover cash from the Sochi Winter Olympics. The GTO is designed to promote a fit and healthy population (ages 6 to 60) ready to defend themselves, their families, and their country.

With 59% of Russia or 86.7 million Russians overweight, citizens will enter competitions in running, swimming, and grenade throwing. An annual report informs the President and the public of Russian fitness.

DUBAI WEIGHT LOSS GOLD

Each year during 30 days of Ramadan fasting, participants receive a gram of gold - $40 USD value in 2019, for each kilogram (2.2 lbs) of weight lost. Participants need to lose at least two kilograms to receive payment. If you're currently eating 4,000 calories a day (average calorie intake for an American), you'll lose 20 pounds over 30 days (4,000-1,500 = 2,500 daily less calories * 7 days = 17,500 calories a week / 3,500 = 5 pounds a week * 4 weeks = 20 pounds) if cut your calorie intake down to 1,500 calories a day. Thru exercising 6 times per week over 4 weeks, you can lose 7 pounds if you burn on average 1,000 calories per workout which JustHuynh Fitness' martial arts and power athletics does. As such you could earn almost $500 USD for losing 12.27 kg (27 pounds) over 4 weeks. That's an excellence reward.

Hussain Nasser Lootah, director general of Dubai Municipality, says "Ramadan is the most appropriate season to launch such initiatives as it reminds us about many health benefits of reducing weight and encourages us to take strong steps to change our bad lifestyles."

LONDON JUNK FOOD AD BAN

In 2018, London Mayor Sadiq Khan banned junk food ads on the London subway tubes and buses in an attempt to reduce childhood obesity. Mayor Khan calls childhood obesity a "ticking time bomb" because 40% of 10-11 year-olds in London are overweight.

Khan along with other city leaders want measures to go from local to national rollout by pressing United Kingdom Prime Minister Theresa May to toughen up its child obesity strategy as there is no national plan to ban junk food advertising seen by children online and during family TV shows.

AUSTRALIA ALCOHOL TAX

In 2018, the Australian Government levied a new tax on alcohol that raises the cost of cask wine by more than 100% to address the nation's growing obesity where 63% of adults and 27% of children are overweight.

LEADERS LEAD BY EXAMPLE

When elected governor of Arkansas in 2003, 300 pound Mike Huckabee was diagnosed with type 2 diabetes and informed by physicians that he would not live more than 10 years if he did not lose weight. Mike was motivated to eat healthier and exercise more when former Governor Frank D. White died from heart attack due to being overweight. He lost over 110 pounds with the "The New York Times" describing the weight loss "as if Mike simply unzipped a fat suit and stepped out."

Since then, Mike declared himself a "recovering foodaholic" and used health care reform as a major focus of his governorship.

PRESIDENTIAL FITNESS

When elections for new heads of states are held for countries around the world, citizens often ask if the prospective leader is "fit to lead" physically, mentally, and emotionally. In the United States, we can compare the current President Donald Trump and his predecessor President Barack Obama's fitness regimen.

When you're President of the United States of America, the whole world is watching. With regards to President Obama's eating habits, the Physicians Committee for Responsible Medicine, a non-profit group, had asked President Obama to stop being photographed eating unhealthy foods such as his love for hot dogs, hamburgers, corn dogs, gumbo, chicken wings, waffles, pancakes, tacos, ice cream, popcorn because 42% of United States' adult population is at risk of being obese by year 2030. Instead advocates recommend President Obama being photographed only when eating healthy foods so people around the world will adopt healthy habits.

President Obama's second weakness is smoking. In 2011, he mentioned the United States making progress with only 46 million Americans addicted to smoking, but tobacco still remains the leading cause of preventable early death. After recently quitting his habit of chewing nicotine gum, President Obama made it a personal mission for tobacco companies to put new warning labels to reduce the smoking population.

To lower the effects of President Obama's desire for unhealthy foods and smoking, his fitness is top notch where he exercises 45 minutes a day for six days a week. One instance of his balancing act was when he followed up a heavy pork chop and beer dinner in Iowa with an early morning hour-long workout to burn off the bad calories. President Obama follows JustHuynh

Fitness' recommendation of combining cardio (Taekwondo) with resistance training for optimal health results.

As for President Donald Trump, he believes that "golf is the only exercise I need because exercising will deplete my energy battery." He made fun of his friends getting knee replacements and hip replacements while he's an injury-free golfer - spending 94 of his 363 first Presidential days at his Trump-branded golf properties. When interviewed at age 71, President Trump revealed his exercise regimen as "I get exercise. I mean I walk, I this, I that...I run over to a building next door."

International inspiration from world leaders should motivate anyone in their professions. In terms of fit world leaders, Canada's Justin Trudeau boxes, China's Xi Jinping dances, France's Emmanuel Macron plays Tennis, and Russia's Vladimir Putin swims, plays hockey, and performs judo.

DEFEAT THE SICKNESS INDUSTRY

Globesity is a word coined by the World Health Organization as "Global Obesity" where 90% of the world will be obese by year 2030 similar to the future displayed in "Wall-E" movie filled with "fitless humans" eating junk food and watching TV.

In order to reduce obesity, sickness industry players such as bad-intentioned pharmaceuticals and insurers must be dealt with. Pharmaceuticals receive large amounts of government taxpayer money for research & development (R&D) for prescription drugs. However, pharmaceuticals are incentivized to provide short-term prescriptions for your health problems so that you, the patient, will endlessly return to buy more drugs. If pharmaceuticals spend R&D money on providing a one-shot cure, then you would be a one-shot customer providing just 1 transaction for pharmaceuticals. With this moral hazard, there must be government pressure on pharmaceuticals to focus on cures instead of temporary prescriptions, but this is no easy feat as pharmaceuticals have a strong lobbyist presence and provide large amounts of political funding contributions. Just like the government tried to discipline greedy Wall Street Bankers who caused the 2008 Subprime Mortgage Financial Crisis by giving out mortgages to anyone with a FICO score and a pulse that left millions of Americans unemployed, bankrupt, and robbed of the American Dream of homeownership, the government must discipline pharmaceuticals to take people's health in their best interest.

The American Healthcare system is one of the most broken in the world where many unhealthy people are refused care by hospitals for not having adequate insurance coverage. Due to the exorbitant premiums required by insurers, some patients end up bankrupt causing the insurers to sell the patients to debt collectors.

To fix a broken system, company leaders must be willing to disrupt the vulturous insurers. In 2018, Jeff Bezos, Warren Buffett, and Jamie Dimon, whose companies have millions of employees, are joining forces to take the lead with their own healthcare plan that could be rolled out nationally.

CHAPTER 14

COACHING

Give a man a fish and you feed him for a day. Teach a man to fish and you feed him for a lifetime

- Lao Tzu

SCHOOL COACHING - LEADERSHIP

The most successful people in the world have coaches to help them thrive in life and business.

When you were in grade school, your classroom teacher whether it be a core subject, foreign language, or music - coached you to class. If you participated in youth sports, your coach provided a workout and gameplan for you to excel during competition.

I appreciated my high school track coach who taught me the benefits of sprinting and how to be a great leader as I captained the team senior year. My other favorite coach was my Karate Sensei who taught me focus, discipline, confidence, and the power of martial arts to defend yourself.

LIFE COACHING - LOVE

As you go thru life and marry the love of your life, you'll start raising a family, buying a home, launching a business, etc.

Your parents or guardians are your life coaches. If you came from a positive upbringing, do not ignore your parents. Since graduating high school, I continue to call my mom every day to provide her life updates and more importantly to let her know that I'm alive. Whether it's personal or professional questions, my parents advise me on difficult situations.

When you get married, your number one friend will be your husband or wife so you must be a great listener to help each other thrive. Studies show that being married to a significant other bolsters your career potential. Successful people like Facebook's Mark Zuckerberg, Kate Spade's Kate Spade, Snap's Evan Spiegel, and Spanx's Sara Blakely all achieved success from being married. When Tesla CEO Elon Musk got dumped by actress Amber Heard, he became lovesick and lonely. You'll notice in 2018 that Elon was active on Twitter bashing stock short sellers such as offering short shorts to billionaire David Einhorn for losing large sums of money for shorting Tesla. This didn't stop as Elon smoked weed on Joe Rogan's podcast and messaged on Twitter that he wanted to take Tesla private at $420 a share - which is a number linked to smoking weed. As such, the Security and Exchanges Commission fined Elon $20 million and asked him to step down as Chairman of Tesla's Board for three years. The presence of a loved one could have helped counsel Elon before these incidences.

BUSINESS COACHING - MENTOR MASTERMIND

Professionally, most can learn from their boss so that they can one day ascend into higher positions. My favorite mentor strategy is that of Napoleon Hill who each night meets with his "Mentor Mastermind" which is an assembly of all the businesspeople that he admires based on their particular success strategies. The top 2 mentors in my "Mentor Mastermind" are Sam Walton of Walmart for his hustle in saying the "Customer is King" and Steve Jobs of Apple for his fearlessness saying "We all eventually die, so operate like you have nothing to lose." This approach allows Steve Jobs to create world-changing premium products that loyal customers happily pay for.

If you're an employee, you must maintain a great relationship with your boss in order to keep your job, advance in the company, and position yourself for a future job switch. If you're a CEO who has raised investor funding, then you must maintain an honest dialogue with your investors about your business performance and challenges. If you fully-own your business, then customers are your boss and you must provide an amazing product and service as customers serve as your coach to solving their problems which they're willing to pay you to solve.

FITNESS CEO & CELEBRITY COACHING

In business or hollywood, the most successful people hire fitness instructors as coaches. 77% of people do not meet the health guidelines of exercising 3 times per week. Those that do exercise mostly plateau as they repeat the same exercises not giving the body muscle confusion for continuous growth. Health is priceless and investing in fitness coaching is the best investment you'll ever make.

If the busiest and richest person in the world Jeff Bezos of Amazon and Queen Elizabeth at Age 92 in 2018 can both stay healthy thru fitness coaches, you can invest time to stay healthy as well. Whether you're looking to lose weight for the beach, get ready for an athletic competition, get slim for a wedding suit or dress, or just to get healthy, reach out to our JustHuynh Fitness' team and we'll coach you to success with martial arts and power athletics.

CHAPTER 15

CONFIDENCE AND MENTAL HEALTH

In the world of business, the people who are most successful are those who are doing what they love...Think about it...Doing what we love is a major contributor to our happiness as humans.

\- Warren Buffett

MENTAL FITNESS - HIKIKOMORI

What is mental health? Mental health includes your emotional, psychological, and social well-being that affects how you think, feel, and act. Greek Philosopher Plato said it best, "In order for man to SUCCEED in life, God provided him with two means, EDUCATION and PHYSICAL ACTIVITY. One for the soul and the other for the body. With these two means, man can attain PERFECTION."

Exercise is the ultimate medicine as a defense against mood swings, Alzheimer's, and ADHD. Exercise allows you to find your "eternal elixir of youth" to enjoy life happily and healthily with your kids, family, and friends.

Unfortunately, 1 in 10 adults in the United States struggles with depression - experiencing disrupted sleep, loss of appetite, forgetfulness, and suicidal thoughts as experienced by recent celebrity suicides by designer Kate Spade (hung herself with a scarf refusing to divorce her husband), foodie Anthony Bourdain (hung himself after seeing pictures of his girlfriend Asia Argento with another man), DJ Avicii (cut himself with broken glass being depressed from pancreatitis where his gallbladder and appendix were removed due to excessive drinking), politician R. Budd Dwyer (shot himself in the mouth live in front of television cameras after being found guilty of bribery charges), CEO Colin Kroll (overdosed on heroin and cocaine after breaking up from a wedding engagement), hedge fund executive Charles Murphy (jumped from 20 stories high after losing $7 billion of client's money in Bernie Madoff's Ponzi scheme), Mac Miller (overdosed after breakup with singer Ariana Grande), and actor Robin Williams.

Mental health issues may arise in all phases of your life: personally if you're going thru a divorce, breakup, or a death in the family, professionally if you've been declined a promotion or suffered huge financial losses, academically if you performed below expectations or got bullied by your classmates, and athletically if you got cut from your team or lost a game.

Tragically in 2018, longtime Hillsborough County Florida deputy sheriff Chad Chronister murdered his 54-year-old wife, 32-year-old daughter, and 6-year-old granddaughter before shooting himself in front of local authorities near his granddaughter's school. Before committing suicide, he had called the local police station saying he was experiencing "financial and health" problems so wanted to kill himself. If you or someone is struggling with depression, call your National Suicide Prevention Lifeline to get help. There is no need to kill innocent people.

In the same year in Tennessee, Cynthia Collier murdered her four adopted Chinese home-schooled children - shooting 14-year-old Bo Li 4 times while in bed, 14-year-old Meigan Lin 8 times while in bed, 15-year-old Lia Lin 9 times while in bed, and 17-year-old Kaileigh Lin 13 times in the bathroom before Cynthia shot herself in the head. Cynthia did not want her separated husband to win legal parenting time with her four adopted Chinese children who he's abandoned for the past nine years. In order to keep her four adopted children from her husband, Cynthia decided to stay together with her four children in heaven by murdering everyone. Please seek help instead of resorting to murder in parental disputes.

In 2018, the World Health Organization classified "gaming disorder" as a mental health condition, stating that problematic gaming behavior might cause problems in other areas of your life. There is a strong connection between videogames and violence especially in the wake of shootings at schools and public places throughout the United States. Many gamers are suffering a problem called "Hikikomori" which is the complete social withdrawal from real life into a virtual life. Gamers miss out on the beauty of nature, loving relationships and satisfaction of contributing to a better world, all for a fake life.

Barriers exist for mental illness treatment where an astonishing 60% of American adults and 50% of children ages 8–15, receive no treatment for their mental illness diagnoses. Treatments like mental health medications and psychotherapy are available but people face a stigma going thru therapy and are afraid of side effects from medication.

Fortunately as Plato mentioned, instead of pills, there is an all-natural treatment called exercise. Depression manifests physically by causing low energy, appetite changes, and body aches.

A Duke University study found that those who exercised at a moderate level 40 minutes three to five times each week experienced the greatest antidepressant effect. Exercise not only increases blood flow to the brain, it releases endorphins - the body's very own natural antidepressant and releases other neurotransmitters like serotonin which lift mood.

Anyone who has raced, competed, fought, or lifted knows first-hand the immediate sense of endorphin-induced euphoria where you feel upbeat and clear-headed. Other important exercise benefits include enhanced mood and energy, reduced stress, deeper relaxation, improved mental clarity, higher self-esteem, and increased spiritual connection. In addition to exercise when you're fighting a negative mindset, seek the social support of family and friends instead of drugs, alcohol, and overeating to improve mental health.

CELEBRITY WEIGHT LOSS TRANSFORMATION

Superheros and Sportstars all have amazing bodies that fans want. When celebrities have babies or start a dad-bod, it only takes a few months to lose - leaving at times jealous. However, celebrities aren't some out-of-this-world creature that have superpowers of weight loss. They're human, just like you and me. Here's a look at the celebrity secrets for weight loss that we share with our JustHuynh Fitness clients for inspiration.

Hard Work and Determination: Celebrities know that workouts are just as important as nutrition. Drew Carey host of the "Price is Right" show had Type 2 diabetes and mentioned "I was tired of health problems and carrying around extra weight. So I cut carbs and hit the gym religiously - dropping 80 pounds to overcome diabetes without medication."

Right Mindset: Most celebrities have goals that they desperately want to achieve such as getting their pre-baby body back. Decide what you want to get out of being healthy, whether it's to lose a certain amount of pounds, drop a few dress sizes, play with your kids, or find love. Tennis Champion Billie Jean King mentioned "As a tennis great, I've always been mindful of diet and exercise. When diagnosed with Type 2 diabetes in 2007, I cut back on carbs and sugars. That's not fun for a lot of people, but it sure is fun to feel good."

Make Exercise a Social Event: publicly share your journey for social accountability and motivation. Age is just a number as Carole Carson proved it's never too late to start being healthy again. At Age 60, Carole publicly admitted shame of being fat in a Nevada local newspaper and documented her journey from fat (butterball) to fit (butterfly) that inspired 1,000 community members to train together with her.

Age is Just a Number: committing to exercise with someone else can help you stick with your fitness routine. Steve Harvey host of "Family Feud" said "My arms were just sitting there and I got tired of looking at myself with piece of meat hanging around. So I hired a trainer to slim down, eat right, and stopped whining about being too old to get in shape."

BOARDROOM & BEDROOM DOMINANCE

People who succeed and dominate the exercise room gain the needed confidence to dominate in the bedroom and boardroom.

By putting in quality time in the exercise room, you now have the ability to "finish" any task you start. Golf has a famous saying of "Drive For Show, Putt For Dough." In fitness, the "dough" is your ability to complete your workout to achieve your fitness goals. The "drive" is your intent.

In terms of mentality, I personally adopt a "Practice like you've never won. Perform like you've never lost" mentality where the practices and workouts are harder than the competition or game itself. Whenever I workout, I raise my performance level to "Super Saiyan" Dragon Ball Z style so that I blow out everyone in a team sport competition due to my speed, power, and endurance. It's a wonderful feeling and you can thrive in life with such a mentality.

You need to stay focused when exercising outside for cardio or inside a gym around other members as there will always be haters who judge you. Just adopt a "Doubt me, Hate me…You're the Inspiration I need" mentality because you can "shut everyone up" by dominating your workout while treating everyone with respect. Such an attitude may even change the hater's personality to appreciate greatness in front of their eyes. It amazes me when people idolize Michael Jordan or Serena Williams because they are untouchable, but when there are amazing athletes in public or gym, people become jealous. Instead haters should walk up to the amazing athlete and ask for tips or just pay attention to what they're doing.

By dominating the exercise room, you'll transform into a person physically with a great body and emotionally with more confidence due to the fact that you can complete the hardest workouts. Whether you're single, in a relationship, or married, the gains from the exercise room will translate over into the bedroom where you'll be more attractive to anyone you like.

Women and men each love to focus on particular parts of their body due to historical standards from the Greek Gods and Hollywood Celebrities. Women love working on their butt and men love working on their chest, arms, and abs. When my wife was choosing a man that she could spend the rest of her life with, she wanted someone who was smart, humble, and strong. By prioritizing fitness, I improved my "smarts" - obtaining degrees from Bowdoin College (#4 ranked liberal arts college in the United States) and Vanderbilt University (#14 ranked university in the United States), developed "humbleness" from martial arts to treat everyone with respect, and "strength" thru JustHuynh Fitness' martial arts and power athletics.

Most people in their teenage and twenties spend those years experimenting on dating sites swiping away on Tinder and Match.com or if you're too busy to find love in your 40s, 50s, 60s, 70s, and 80s, you might marry a significant other with a bigger than normal age difference - being labelled a Sugar Daddy (i.e. Hugh Hefner at age 86 married a 26 year old women, Robert Duvall at age 74 married a 33 year old women, Rupert Murdoch at age 68 married a 30 year old women, Harrison Ford at age 68 married a 46 year old women, Clint Eastwood at age 66 married a 31 year old women, Steve Martin at age 62 married a 36 year old women, Donald Trump at age 58 married a 34 year old women, Alec Baldwin at age 53 married a 27 year old women) or Sugar Mommy (Brigitte Trogneux at age 53 married her high school student and now French President Emmanuel Macron when he was 29, Demi Moore at age 43 married a 28 year old man). That's fine.

Whatever your love journey despite any large age differences, having a significant other is important in life as Napoleon Hill mentions that "Sexual expression is the strongest human emotion that when transmuted and harnessed into action may raise your status to genius. Achievement building genius is obtained thru the eternal triangle of love, sex, and romance for the magnetism benefits (handshake, voice, posture, thought, appearance) in how you carry yourself." Success stories by tech titans Mark Zuckerberg of Facebook and Evan Spiegel of Snap prove that locking down love has accelerated their career than being single.

Married, my wife has been supportive on JustHuynh Fitness' mission to help the 2 billion overweight people get healthy thru martial arts and power athletic. Entrepreneurship is not easy as you can only succeed if you're passionate about the problem and customers love your product.

As a professional, being fit helps you dominate the boardroom to attain bonuses, promotions, and high-profile assignments. As an entrepreneur, you'll close more sales and recruit a strong team.

FEAR IS JUST A STATE OF MIND

My fitness passion and leadership talents weren't being put to use for the betterment of the world sitting in a cubicle in a 9-5 job. So in the summer of 2016 after completing my MBA from Vanderbilt and getting married, my wife supported me in pursuing my passion for global health thru JustHuynh Fitness to reject 6 figure career opportunities with the FBI and Samsung.

For me, most humbling was when I went from a $62.50 an hour MBA corporate job offer to making $8 an hour driving Uber. While building up JustHuynh Fitness' brand in Boston as quickly as possible to surpass my forfeited MBA salary in order to have kids, I applied for part-time positions but my MBA and startup experience was deemed overqualified by human resource recruiters who couldn't afford my talent and experience level especially with many of their CEOs being similar age.

Remember fear is just a state of mind especially in times when no one helps you during times of struggle including your family, friends, and significant others. To succeed, you have to be able to put your foot on the neck of fear to not worry about what the naysayers think, say, or do.

Even though I made less money right away compared to an MBA 6 figure salary, I was willing to exchange that so I could wake-up everyday able to provide for my family and pursue my passion of helping the 2 billion overweight people get healthy. The numerous fitness challenges overcome helped me mentally as an entrepreneur to navigate the darkest times such as moments of depression when my parents, who I've called everyday since college, ask if I've surpassed my MBA salary yet or when I will have children as I'm now age 30. Asian parents have high standards for their children to achieve the best grades in high school and scores on the college entrance exams to get into the best universities that lead to high-paying jobs and a wonderful wife or husband. I made it all the way to a 6 figure job offer and disappointed my parents by passing up on Samsung and the FBI, but they are now supportive of entrepreneurship despite my high education level.

In life, I've been a trailblazer in my family as my goal is to break the "bamboo ceiling" where Asians are quiet, nerdy, submissive, and weak. Having been on both sides of the weight spectrum where I was a skinny weak kid and then a fat clumsy kid, I've experienced my fair share of bullying based on my physique, color of my skin, and demeanor. Fitness changed everything and I hope to empower everyone to achieve the best body they can so that they can achieve anything they want in life.

In business, being FIT is a LEAD MAGNET, I love helping other entrepreneurs realize that staying fit should be a top priority since health is our most important asset. If you don't have your health, you won't be able to enjoy any wealth that you have with those you love. Business is an endurance sport, and the CEOs who can best lead their companies to success are those who stay healthy, strong and active. One of favorite mantras is "Your smile is your logo, your personality is your business card, how you leave others feeling after an experience with you becomes your trademark." By being fit and passionately pursuing your career, people will enjoy the value you provide.

I had many epic moments at Vanderbilt Business School, but the one I remember the most is when my team of 4 were the only 1st year MBAs in a class of 30 other 2nd year students. In the second semester for 2nd year students, most students have already locked down a six figure job so are just showing up to pass the class and are not as engaged with the class material. The lack of class enthusiasm didn't deter me from participating in class discussions to learn as much as possible especially on topics relating to doing business in China. When the final presentation came and the professor asked which order teams wanted to present, I enthusiastically raised my hand to go first as I love setting the standard. Our professor agreed, but threw in a caveat by putting a bounty for the class to "break my leg" before the presentation as I was too confident and would dominate. They laughed and we got the highest grades in the class. Even though we were the only 1st year MBAs in the class, there is no need to fear the 2nd year students as long as you present expertly on your topic.

Reddit co-founder Alex Ohanian, husband of tennis superstar Serena Williams, during his 100 university nationwide tour promoting his book "Without Their Permission," shares his story overcoming fear of rejection when Yahoo executives didn't take Reddit seriously in a potential acquisition. Yahoo said "Reddit's website visitor count is a rounding error compared to ours." Not shaken and to overcome rejection, Alex says "There are always going to be haters in our lives. The best thing we can do is use their criticism for ammunition. Create your own "wall of negative reinforcement" that features printouts of commentary from haters. Any time I need motivation, I can look over to the wall and see someone who I wanted to prove wrong. For Yahoo, I printed "You are a rounding error" on the wall."

Life is too short to be stuck in fear. Instead use haters and challenges as motivation to prove everyone wrong and yourself that "anything is possible."

CHAPTER 16

Habitual Commitment

I shall be telling this with a sigh. Somewhere ages and ages hence. Two roads diverged in a wood, and I - I took the one less travelled by and that has made all the difference

- Robert Frost

MOTIVATION TO EXERCISE

Exercise may feel boring, but your time investment with fitness is for the benefits such as increased intelligence, self defense skills, love life, and health to enjoy time with your family and friends.

In life, you may run into situations where you're being assessed by someone else such as: Who to ADMIT or REJECT? (College or Business School), Who to pick on ALL-STAR TEAM? (Work or School Project), Who to HIRE or FIRE? (Staffing Decisions), Who to PROMOTE or DEMOTE? (Talent Evaluations), Who's life to SAVE or PULL PLUG ON? (Medical Resource Constraints), Who is the #1 Pick or UNDRAFTED? (Team Sports), Who to DATE, MARRY, DUMP? (Love).

Being fit helps you thrive personally and professionally. Knowing this, you should be addicted with being fit.

Motivation Wall: similar to your childhood days when you hung posters of idols who you wanted to become, use that same motivation wall for your fitness goals. Place a picture of your best current self in between 2 people that inspire you and post on a wall so you can see everyday for motivation. For me, I have Dragon Ball Z Super Saiyan Goku as he channels insane amounts of energy thru anger to conquer challenges which I use during my fighting, pick-up sports, and sprinting. As a martial artist, my second idol is Bruce Lee as he is fearless and master of mind games.

Success Mindset: when the going gets tough, you want to embrace a success mindset to eliminate thoughts of failure while working out. Envisioning success helps you attack your fitness with confidence. Rewatch any successful picture or video of you before your workout. As a short Asian,

I've always been counted out so rewatch the comeback track relay victory against the younger students during business school and re-enact my victory against a 2nd degree black belt to cultivate a winning and fearless attitude.

Action Movies: when you feel in a rut, go to the movie theatres or watch any movie starring Tom Cruise, Gal Gadot, Jackie Chan, Jennifer Lawrence, Rocky, etc to bring that inner-hero mode out.

Travel: with over 7 billion people in the world, it helps to get out of your city to see what life is like. Travelling to Rio de Janeiro right before the 2014 World Cup opened my eyes as everyone from children to retirees are fit due to embracement of soccer and beach sports. Then take a flight to Dallas, Texas where "Everything is Bigger in Texas" where you'll see many overweight people eating out of control and refusing to exercise. It's a sad sight that JustHuynh Fitness will help with our studios and online training programs. By travelling, you'll get to see the impact being fit (Rio) vs unfit (Dallas) has on people's lives.

Public: At Age 60, Carole Carson, who wrote the book "From Fat to Fit," went public with her Nevada community about her 12 week transformation journey from "fat to fit" as she was very ashamed of not prioritizing health. She went public as a way to keep accountable to her goals. Carole's successful completion of her health goals inspired thousands of others to pursue "fat to fit" transformations of their own. You too can go public with local reporters to inspire your community to get fit.

Bet Against Friends: You can pay friends a monetary penalty for skipping workouts. It's up to you to be honest.

Charity Commitment Contract: Choose a charity that you hate and an amount that you must donate if you fail to finish your workout plan. Be honest and make payment to the disliked charity if you miss your workout.

MENTAL PREPARATION TO EXERCISE

Hollywood and Sports are the best source of inspiration to unlock your max potential.

Next Level Performance: Wonder Woman is a great role model for her ability to channel anger thru love to increase her power when fighting off villains. Similarly, Dragon Ball Z's Goku channels super-power thru anger. You can use anger from haters or enemies to push beyond your fitness levels.

Adrenaline Rush: Channeling Tom Cruise in Mission Impossible, Jackie Chan in Rush Hour, or James Bond pushes you to workout as if you're fighting to survive.

Comeback Victory: Sports Legends such as Tom Brady, Serena Williams, and Michael Jordan are famous for overcoming deficits to will their teams to victory. Having the confidence of a legend can push you thru any self doubts in a workout or fitness journey.

Chip on Shoulder: Everyone including the most successful people in the world have experienced rejection. Whether it's being turned down by a girl or guy you had a crush on, being picked last or not being picked at all during your childhood recess soccer game, being rejected from your dream college, being rejected from your dream job, not getting promoted over a less qualified co-worker due to them playing office politics better, etc. The best channel these rejections as motivation to show the doubters and haters that they underestimated you.

Feeling Sexy: Like Channing Tatum in Magic Mike or any Hollywood Actress starring in a sexy movie, embracing your sexiness helps you attain your physical goals to improve your personal love life.

FITNESS GEAR FOR CONFIDENCE

There are many gyms to choose from. As a gym member investing money to workout there, don't let people hold you back from greatness.

Gear: Amazing gear paired with confidence will have the gym respecting your dedication so you can focus on your workout. JustHuynh Fitness has gear with motivational quotes on the back that will leave other gym goers respecting your confidence. My favorite shirt says "Forget haters who talk behind your back. They're behind you for a reason." Every time a gym goer gets a chance to connect eyes with me they are either in awe or fear which accomplishes my mission of training confidently.

Personal Brand: As you get better physically, you'll start developing a personal brand at work, in public, at home, and in the gym. Having transformed from fat to fit, I've developed a reputation as franchise (my nickname), special agent (speed), super saiyan (martial arts), 444am (my wakeup time), the closer (presentation skills), and ninja (quick personality).

MUSIC TO EXERCISE - SAMPLE PLAYLIST

Having a great music playlist helps you perform at a higher level like you see athletes wearing headphones during individual practices or fitness studios blasting fast beat music. Electronic Music such as from Tiesto or Steve Aoki, Club Remixes of top hip-hop hits, and Korean Pop will help you let loose. Research has found that high tempo music like hip hop can create strong arousal and performance readiness. Other evidence finds the intensity of the emotional response can linger long after the music has stopped. After a great workout, you will be hyped for the remainder of your day to excel personally and professionally.

Here is a 30 song playlist that can get you thru a workout: "Remember the Name" by Fort Minor, "Shape of You" by Ed Sheeran, "End Game" by Taylor Swift, "Let's Go" by Calvin Harris, "Sucker for Pain" by Lil Wayne, "No Brainer" by DJ Khaled ft Justin Bieber, "Work" by Rihanna ft Drake, "One Dance" by Drake, "Jackie Chan" by Tiesto, "Sorry Not Sorry" by Demi Lovato, "Sexy Bitch" by David Guetta ft Akon, "Hello Friday" by Flo Rida ft Jason Derulo, "Beat It" by Michael Jackson, "Havana" by Camila Cabello, "Champion" by Kanye West, "Give Me Everything" by Pitbull, "Lose Yourself" by Eminem, "Sexy and I Know It" by LMFAO, "A Star is Born" by Jay-Z ft J. Cole, "Taki Taki" by DJ Snake, "Finesse" by Bruno Mars ft Cardi B, "Moneymaker" by Ludacris ft Pharrell, "Wild One" by Flo Rida ft Sia, "Despacito" by Luis Fonsi, "Lose Control" by Missy Elliott ft Ciara, "Turn Down For What" by DJ Snake, "Forever" by Drake, "Kill Em With Kindness" by Selena Gomez, "How Deep is Your Love" by Calvin Harris ft Disciples, and "Eye of the Tiger" by Survivor.

HOME GYM EQUIPMENT

The future of fitness is in-home where you can set-up a basic gym in your home or apartment and hire a fitness instructor (online, virtual, or in-person) to help you exercise in the comfort of your home. JustHuynh Fitness highly recommends client attend a fitness studio for cardio days and exercise at home during weight lifting days. If there is no local fitness studio of your choice nearby, you can purchase an in-home treadmill and kickboxing bag to perform the cardio workout with an online training program that JustHuynh Fitness offers.

As of 2017, there are 55 million people in the United States with gym memberships and only 20% or 11 million people actually go to the gym. That means there are over 300 million people in the United States who choose the couch over the gym resulting in only 23% of Americans meeting the World Health Organization's guideline of exercising 3 times per week.

All you need is a bench press setup with barbells and weight plates, dumbbells, and recovery equipment such as a hamstring foam roller and resistance bands. Instead of being judged inside a gym during weight lifting days, you can lift weights in a comfortable environment in your home.

CHOOSING A GYM

Choose a gym for access to equipment that you don't have available at home for non-martial arts training days such as a swimming pool, outdoor track, and weight lifting machines.

In selecting gyms, my favorite is the YMCA as it's a family friendly judgement-free zone and allows members to use gyms anywhere in the world that is a huge convenience when you are travelling away from home.

Surprisingly, 80% of 55 million Americans with gym members don't use their paying gym membership. Start being proactive with your health by using your gym membership for weight lifting or non-martial arts workouts.

SHARING ECONOMY

We live in an era where people are now comfortable sharing time with strangers who may eventually become friends such as ridesharing (Uber, Lyft), lodging (AirBnB), dating (Tinder, Bumble), dog walking (Wag), game playing (Fortnite), and social networks (Facebook, Instagram).

In social settings, people may experience AVE (Abstinence Violation Effect) where people hide from their support group when they FAIL to meet the group's expectations, instead of turning to the group for help. You see this happen all the time in families, classrooms, sports teams, business groups, etc. You must view failure as a stepping stone to greatness.

Experiences are moments that you'll always treasure. With fitness, working out together with other community members in a studio or sharing the online fitness training program journey together provides the needed social accountability and motivation for you to achieve your fitness goals.

FITNESS MONEY WASTERS

JustHuynh Fitness' studio group fitness classes are around $30 each, personal training around $95 per session, and online training programs around $100 per month.

People are willing to pay $200,000 for a private golf lesson with Tiger Woods, $2,000 to watch high profile sports games, $100 a week on coffee, and many random purchases that have no benefit for their mental, physical, or financial wellness.

Based on my experience attending college from years 2006-2010 at Bowdoin College in my home state of Maine, the average American college student spent $200,000 on a 4 year education which averages out at $240 for a 1-hour class. Most of us are proud of our college education.

You should also be proud of investing in your health thru fitness programs that will bring a huge return on investment for your health, life, and career. Reduce your weekly spending on coffee, alcohol, drugs, fast food, dining out, and unneeded shopping for better health and saved money.

CHAPTER 17

90 DAY FITNESS TRANSFORMATION

The weak die out and the strong survive, and will live on forever

- Anne Frank

CALORIE BURN & FAT LOSS 12 WEEK MATH

Per most doctor's expert opinion, people on average should eat 2,000 calories a day to maintain weight and reduce to a safe 1,500 calories per day to lose one pound a week. Mathematically by dropping 500 calories a day or 3,500 calories weekly - you can lose one pound. However, not everyone starts out at a current daily calorie intake of 2,000. The average American consumes 3,770 calories and overweight consume 6,700 calories a day. On an interesting note, Olympic Swimmer Michael Phelps famously consumed 10,000 calories a day during his 2018 8 Olympic Gold Medal run as he burned so many calories from swimming. So for the average person cutting from 3,770 to 1,500 calories per day that is a 2,270 daily calorie reduction or 15,890 per week which is 4.54 pounds lost per week. The overweight dropping from 6,700 to 1,500 calories per day will reduce weekly calories by 36,400 which is 10.4 pounds lost per week.

If you exercise for 45-60 minutes 6 times per week, you will burn 1,200 calories each day (1,000 from workout and 200 from afterburn), totalling 7,200 calories each week or 2 pounds loss per week.

With the goal of exercising 45-60 minutes 6 times per week and a 1,500 daily calorie nutrition, here is how much weight you may lose if stay dedicated over 12 weeks.

If you're currently someone who is consuming 2,000 calories per day, you may lose 2 pound per week and 24 pounds over 12 weeks. If you're currently consuming 3,770 calories per day, you may lose 6.54 pounds per week and 78.48 pounds over 12 weeks. If you're overweight consuming 6,700 calories per day, you may lose 12.4 pounds per week and 148.8 pounds over 12 weeks. Based on your situation, you can approach your next 12 week fitness transformation journey with these realistic weight loss goals in mind.

DIABETES & OBESITY PREVENTION

As of 2018, there are over 300 million people worldwide with diabetes. Fortunately 90% are Type 2 who can improve thru nutrition and exercise. Per leading health experts, losing 7% of your total weight over 12 weeks can improve your insulin performance by 57% that can help reduce your medication dependence.

Each week over the next 12 weeks, perform 3 cardio and 3 weight lifting sessions. For example you can perform weight lifting on Monday, Wednesday, and Friday then do cardio on Tuesday, Thursday, and Saturday - taking Sunday off to rest, enjoy, and let the body transform. Women don't need to be worried about bulking up as women don't have the testosterone levels of men that promote bulky muscles. Weight lifting helps open up muscle cells for glucose to escape the bloodstream to reduce diabetes risk.

Remember to warm-up before your workout and recover as needed for maximum gains.

CARDIO WORKOUTS

Keep you cardio sessions to 45-60 minutes a day. You can sprint on the track or treadmill, swim, perform martial arts, play team sports like soccer or basketball, play heads up sports like squash or tennis, row, or bike. Change up your routine from time to time and you won't get bored.

JustHuynh Fitness' martial arts online program is the best cardio 3 times per week that you can perform with a freestanding or hanging kickboxing bag. You can also join a local JustHuynh Fitness studio or reach out to us if you're interested in opening up a studio as a licensee in your city.

WEIGHT LIFTING WORKOUTS

Lifting weights you want to keep your session to 45 minutes. The most popular format is performing 10 reps of an exercise with great form - often working hard on reps 9 and 10 or else the weight is too light. Arnold Schwarzenegger famously said that "the last 3 or 4 reps is what makes the muscle grow. This area of pain divides the champion from someone else who is not a champion." Remember that. With weight lifting you definitely want to mix up your exercises for muscle confusion. To start, spend one day on chest and triceps, a second day on biceps and back, and third day on shoulders and forearms. Never forget legs so include a couple leg exercises during each of your weight lifting days.

Before performing weights, JustHuynh Fitness recommends that you perform 20-30 minutes of high intensity speed work on the track or treadmill. Warm up with an 800 meter run at 75% of your max mile time. Then perform any of the following speed workouts with full recovery in between. When you're recovering, be active by performing air jump ropes, abs, or air punching drills. For sprinting you can perform 10 100 meter sprints, 8 200 meter sprints, 3 300 meter sprints, 3 400 meter sprints, or a ladder workout consisting of 200 meter/300 meter/400 meter/300 meter/200 meter sprints.

WEEKLY WORKOUT PLAN

To achieve an "Ageless Athletic Assassin," develop a weekly healthy habit of strength training 3 days a week and martial arts 3 days a week with JustHuynh Fitness' online training program at www.justhuynh.com.

Below is sample weekly workout plan for strength training days that you can easily do with in-home gym equipment, in your hotel gym or at your local gym. If you're working out in a hotel gym that doesn't have a barbell, weight plates, or kettlebells, use dumbbells. You can never forget legs so leg exercises are included in each of the strength training days. You will also start each workout with sprint training to get faster and warmed up before you lift. During recovery periods between the run or sprints, perform jump ropes or punching variations such as left/right punches to the head, hook punches to the jaw, uppercut punches to the chin, palm strikes to the nose, and inward elbow strikes to the jaw. There will be 3 superset workouts meaning you perform all exercises in the superset straight thru without rest and you'll rest for 30 seconds after each superset. To get the best results, focus on form - performing the exercise at a controlled speed. The last 2-3 reps of a set should always be hard to finish. If not, increase the weight. If you can't get to those last 2-3 reps, decrease the weight. The goal is to get stronger, faster, and injury free. Reward yourself with one day off a week either on Saturday or Sunday.

Strength Training Day 1 (Chest, Triceps): 1 mile run at 90% of your 1 mile time. Perform 4 200 meter sprints 90% max speed of your 200 meter time...Superset 1: Barbell Flat Bench Chest Press (2x10), Triceps Bench Dips (2x15), Bulgarian Split Squats (2x10 Each Side), Flat Bench Dumbbell Pull-Over (2x10), Standing 1-Arm Overhead Tricep Extension (2x10 each side), Barbell Full Squats (2x10)...Superset 2: Incline Dumbbell Chest Flyes (2x15), Close-Grip Flat Bench Barbell Chest Press (2x10), Sumo Squat with

Dumbbell (2x10), Neutral Grip Flat Bench Dumbbell Chest Press (2x12), Diamond Pushups (2x15), Step Ups on Bench (2x20 each side)...Superset 3: Incline Barbell Bench Chest Press (2x10), Flat Bench Dumbbell Skull Crushers (2x15), Standing Barbell Calf Raise (2x20), Pushups (2x30), Neutral Grip Pull-ups (2x10), Lunge Pulses (2x20 each side)

Martial Arts Day 1: online training program or studio classes with JustHuynh Fitness. www.justhuynh.com

Strength Training Day 2 (Bicep, Back): 800 meter run at faster pace than your 1 mile time. Perform 3 400 meter sprints at faster pace than your 800 meter time...Superset 1: Dumbbell Concentration Bicep Curl (2x12 Each side), Bent Over Dumbbell Reverse Fly (2x10), Seal Jacks (2x20), Chinups (2x10), Dumbbell Bent Over Single Arm Row (2x10 Each Side), Jump Rope (2x100)...Superset 2: Hammer Dumbbell Curl (2x10 Each side), Dumbbell High Pull (2x12), Barbell Hip Thrust (2x10), Close Grip Pushup (2x20), Dumbbell Neutral Grip Deadlift (2x10), Dumbbell Jump Squat (2x15)...Superset 3: Reverse Dumbbell Curl (2x12 Each Side), Dumbbell Renegade Rows (2x8 each side), Burpees (2x15), Preacher Dumbbell Curl on Incline Bench (2x12 Each Side), Wide-Grip Pullups (2x5), Reverse Lunge to High Knee (2x10 each side)

Martial Arts Day 2: online training program or studio classes with JustHuynh Fitness. www.justhuynh.com

Strength Training Day 3 (Shoulder, Forearms): 400 meter run at faster pace than your best 800 meter time. Perform 2 300 meter sprints at faster pace than your best 400 meter time. Perform 2 200 meter sprints 90% max speed of your best 200 meter time...Superset 1: Side Dumbbell Lateral Raise (2x10), Dumbbell Farmer's Carry (2x20 seconds), Bench Jumps (2x10), Dumbbell Shoulder Shrugs (2x12), Dumbbell Shoulder Circle Big to Small Rotation (2x20 Each Direction), Kettlebell Swing (2x15)...Superset 2: Leaning Away Dumbbell Lateral Raise (2x10 Each side), Crab Walk (2x20 seconds), Dumbbell Wrist Curls (2x20), Barbell Split Squat (2x8 Each Side), Sitting Dumbbell Shoulder Press (2x10), 180 Degree Dumbbell Wrist Side Rotations (2x20), Barbell Clean and Press (2x10)...Superset 3: Dumbbell Neutral Grip Front Raise (2x10 Each side), Circle Crawl (2x10 Each Direction), Single Leg Toe Touch (2x10 Each side), Dumbbell Seated L-lateral Raise (2x10), Forearm Blaster Stick Roll (2x Roll-until-burn Each direction), Dumbbell Skier Swing (2x20)

Martial Arts Day 3: online training program or studio classes with JustHuynh Fitness. www.justhuynh.com

PART III

AGELESS (SUPERCENTENARIAN)

When you cease to dream, you cease to live

- Malcolm Forbes

CHAPTER 18

DECADES OF DOMINANT AGEING AND LIFE

In the end, it's not the years in your life that count. It's the life in your years

- Abraham Lincoln

AGE IS JUST A NUMBER

"Look good - feel good." This isn't a phrase reserved for just hollywood. Anyone can obtain the Elixir of Youth. Companies are devoting billions of dollars into anti-aging research to slow down the ageing process. Looking young, fit, and smart is the greatest feeling. Who doesn't want that?

We were all put on Earth thru our biological parent's sperms and eggs. You should feel blessed to be alive and remember to treat everyone with respect. In society, many old people despise the young because they are rebels and stronger - like Mark Zuckerberg, Steve Jobs, and Bill Gates. I see this often in the gym when older people complain to the gym managers that I "workout too hard" and make them look bad. I respond to the older person that every person has their physical limits and should never hold back anyone pursuing greatness. You wouldn't ever tell Michael Jordan, Serena Williams, Tom Brady, or Naomi Osaka to "take it easy" in their workouts. With that type of mentality, the young would never become world champions.

Older people must remember that they too were once young and should encourage the young to continue their work ethic as they age for success. In the corporate world with business leaders focused on getting the most out of talent, people keep their jobs based on merits not tenure. You're only valuable based on what you can do today and tomorrow for your company despite your past accomplishments. If there is a younger, hungrier, and cheaper talent option available, business leaders will not hesitate to replace the less-driven lower-performing older talent with the young talent. In sports, older players such as Derek Jeter in baseball, Peyton Manning in football, Kobe Bryant in basketball, Michael Phelps in swimming, and countless others all knew it was time to retire as they could no longer compete at a high level with younger talent able to beat them.

In business, companies like Uber will "deactivate" you as an independent contractor if you have low customer reviews, Amazon will fire their $15-an-hour warehouse employees who use up their "three strikes" policy, IBM has fired 20,000 salaried employees older than age 40 in the last six years in a "rank and yank" system if employees skills are no longer sufficient for their role, and entrepreneurs or small businesses close business if they fail to deliver value to their customers over the competition.

On the other end, younger people should respect their elders as the "young will eventually become old" and your disrespectful attitude toward elders will come back to bite you when you're an elder and younger people make fun of you. People between ages 18-21 are most rebellious during their college years, but they must remember that the world is much bigger than the "college bubble" they currently live in. When they graduate, college students will have to work for a living, find a love partner, and search for their purpose of what they want their legacy to be when they die. These are points college students should think about sooner than later by learning from those who came before them. Too many times when life isn't as enjoyable in college where you can play games, party, sleep in class, or nap, young adults commit suicide because they don't know what to do with their lives after school.

Growing up, everyone had or still have role models whether its Michael Jordan in sports, Taylor Swift in music, Barack Obama in politics, Angelina Jolie in movies, Steve Jobs in business, Oprah Winfrey in television, etc. To live your best life, you must study successful people who came before you so you can set yourself up to win as you age.

FITNESS EXCUSES THRU AGE 70

As you get older, you will enter different phases of life that might hold you back from fitness. During childhood, many children tend to waste their time on social media, video games, and watching TV. In college, students fall into peer pressure to "be cool" by adopting bad habits such as drinking alcohol, smoking cigarettes, taking drugs, and eating junk food. After graduation when you're 21 years old, a quarter centuries worth of bad habits could be killer and leave you susceptible to diabetes and cancer. In your 20s, you're figuring out who you are as a person trying to find potential love partners thru "swiping apps" such as Tinder, dance clubs, work, public encounters, etc. Professionally, you might even be in an industry that has nothing to do with your 4-year $300,000 college education. This is a time period where many people in their twenties "let themselves go" - becoming stressed out with larger waist sizes than ever before. Your 30s and 40s are when you get married and start a family. After having kids, moms are occupied taking care of the children and dads develop a "dad bod" by increasing their alcohol and fast food consumption. In your 50s and 60s, you're at the point in life where you'll experience an "empty nest" at home from children who move out of the home to live at college. Professionally, succession talks are in place as you retire so you're busy ensuring everything is set with your retirement savings and business exit.

Once you hit your 70s, this is the decade where the average human dies. Thinking that your life is no longer how many years or months, but just days or minutes left, you want to pursue all of your "bucket list" items such as travelling to a particular country, hiking a tough mountain, etc. You've already put aside fitness for over seventy years of your life so why start now right? Wrong, you can live past 70 by exercising to age gracefully.

SLOW AGEING WITH EXERCISE - TELOMERES

Per Dr. Jordan Metzl, sports medicine physician at the Hospital for Special Surgery, cardiovascular disease and diabetes are the most expensive diseases in the United States - America spends more than $200 billion per year treating these diseases and their complications. With over 400 million people worldwide with diabetes, experts estimate that diabetes speeds up the aging process by 33% - damaging the body from the inside out. Excess blood sugar destroys blood vessels resulting in wrinkling of skin to more severe effects such as heart disease, blindness, stroke, leg amputations, and Alzheimer's. Rather than pay huge sums for disease treatment, we should be encouraging our patients and communities to be active and exercise daily. Exercise should become a daily habit just like brushing your teeth everyday.

If you want beautiful soft skin instead of the wrinkles that tend to appear as you get older, people who exercise have skin that look ten to twenty years younger than their actual age. Beautiful skin has to do with collagen, a connective tissue between skin and muscle. Exercise boosts collagen production to keep your skin firm, while preserving healthy levels of cortisol, a primary stress hormone, to reduce sebum and fight off pimples. Also, too much alcohol dehydrates your skin and dilates your blood vessels.

For fad diet fanatics, repeatedly gaining and losing weight can stretch the skin and make it sag. Instead make a lifestyle change by getting your macronutrients and healthy calories.

Inside the body as we age, our cell renewal process slows down. Telomeres are an essential part of the repetitive DNA which protects the end of chromosomes from deterioration sort of like having a strong plastic end to your shoelace. Telomeres become shorter as you get older and longer telomeres are associated with longevity. After adjusting for smoking, obesity, alcohol use, gender, race and other factors, Larry Tucker of BYU found in his study that people who exercised the most had significantly longer telomeres than those who were couch potatoes. The most sedentary people had 140 fewer base pairs of DNA at the ends of their telomeres, compared to the most active - a difference of about nine years of cellular aging.

People who did vigorous exercise - at least 5 days of exercise a week, had telomeres that signaled about seven fewer years of biological aging compared to people who did moderate levels of activity. If you love life and want to live longer to accomplish all of your dreams, start exercising.

EXERCISE PROS - SEX, BRAIN, MOOD, HEART

Brain: exercise provides increased blood flow to keep brain cells healthy that fight off Alzheimer's, Parkinson's and other neurodegenerative diseases. When the University of Minnesota followed 2,700 men and women for over 25 years, those who played sports in their teenage years scored better on mental tests when they reached their fifties.

Sex drive: exercise improves blood flow all over your body, including below the belt. "This extra blood surge makes you feel more responsive and aroused" says Mary Jane Minkin - clinical professor of obstetrics and gynecology at Yale School of Medicine. If you watched Netflix's "Haunted in Hill House," Theo lost all sense of feeling until she had sex as her exercise to feel her body again.

Posture: you lose muscle and bone density as you age. Incorporating strength training builds muscle and bone health so you can stand taller.

Mood: exercise produces endorphins such as serotonin and dopamine that puts you in a good mood called a "runner's high."

Heart health: your heart gets weak with inactivity so the heart has to work harder to pump blood throughout your body. Exercise makes your heart stronger to pump oxygen-rich blood efficiently thru your body so you lower your susceptibility to high blood pressure and heart attacks.

Restful sleep: restful sleep is like a fountain of youth. Exercise helps you fall asleep easier to experience deep REM sleep that lowers your stress.

Metabolism: metabolism naturally slows as you age, so it's harder to burn calories. Thru exercise, you'll burn more calories than if you sat on the couch. Resistance training using weights will help you even more as you'll build muscles that fuel greater calorie burn.

LAND OF OPPORTUNITY - JOBS ACT TITLE III

When President Obama signed the Jobs Act Title III, he said "America is a Nation of doers, where visionary founders, who may be the next Bill Gates, Steve Jobs, or Mark Zuckerberg, turn improbable ideas into strong businesses." Only in America can someone pursue their passions freely. If you live in a Nation that promotes free enterprise - take advantage.

Being fit allows you to unlock untapped potential to achieve greatness with new personal heights of mind and body. Never again take living in America or your business-friendly country for granted. Take matters into your own hand as successful people prioritize fitness.

PURSUE YOUR DREAMS TODAY

In addition to providing inspiration on how you're never too old to exercise, you are also never too old to pursue your dreams. It doesn't matter whether you are the President of the United States of America or the CEO of the most valuable company in the world, everyone has the same 24 hours in a day. How you spend those 24 hours is the difference between reaching your goals or not. If you're still in a job that you hate and have an entrepreneurial itch, work your 9AM to 5PM job and get your 6 to 8 hours of beauty sleep - leaving you with 8-10 hours remaining of your 24 hour day. Use those remaining hours to create content and products that overcome your unhappiness with life so you can start living life purposefully providing a solution for customers willing to pay for your service or product. Stop complaining and start doing.

Success can take on many meanings whether it's in your love life, academic achievements, athletic milestones, or business success. Hollywood and athlete success inspire people to pursue their passions. Athletes on average make $20 million a year over a 20 year career that nets them $400 million in their lifetime. Actors like Dwayne Johnson make at least $20 million per movie and singers like Taylor Swift can make $346 million in 53 shows such as she did with her 2018 "Reputation" Tour.

Being fit and healthy allows you to enjoy life. Personally, you can find a compatible love partner and raise a family in your dream house. In college, you'll thrive intellectually to get admitted to elite colleges, obtain the best grades; win club board, captain, or leadership positions; and land lucrative career opportunities over your peers. In business, being fit allows you to get the best assignments, coveted promotions, salary raises, and recognition as a star in the company.

There is no participation trophy in life. You have to put in the work. Just like in sports - teams pick players to serve as stars, starters, role players, and bench warmers. Anyone else doesn't make the team.

To inspire both men and women, we will now review men and women who dominated fitness and business in respective decades of life.

TEENAGE STRIPPER TO SUPERSTARS

Cardi B turned from stripper to superstar. At age 19 needing money to make ends meet, Cardi B was praised that her physique could help her earn more money working as a stripper at the New York Dolls Club from 8pm to 4am Monday through Sunday. Each night, Cardi B paid $100-130 in "house fees" for the right to dance. Depending on the clientele and how busy the club was, she made up to $2,500 a night. With an initial plan to retire from stripping at 25, Cardi B quit stripping at age 22 - having become a hit on Instagram after paying for plastic surgeries on her boob and butt. Cardi B broke out as a global superstar when she dethroned Taylor Swift to top the Billboard Hot 100, becoming only the second female rapper to ever score a chart topping solo song after Lauryn Hill did so in 1998.

For fitness, Cardi's been working out twice a day as she wants to get an amazing body for public appearance like the BETs in 2017.

Like teenage sensation Cardi B, Channing Tatum also transformed from stripper to superstar. At age 19, Channing was an athletic boy who dropped out of the University of South Florida despite his football scholarship. Stripping in Tampa Bay Florida was his post-high school career choice as he wanted to continue partying, drinking, and living a wild lifestyle.

After having success in Hollywood, someone leaked a video of Channing as a stripper. Rather than hide, Channing morphed what could have been the most embarrassing chapter of his past into the cornerstone of his present with the movie "Magic Mike" and launched a "Magic Mike" show at Casinos as well.

To carve a "Magic Mike" body, Channing prioritizes the Iron Man sports. He'd bike for 20 miles in the morning, then do 5 water burpees (lap in a pool, jump out of the water, 10 sit-ups, jump back in for another lap), hit the weights (shoulder presses, squats, chest bench presses), and run 4 sets of intervals on the treadmill (run 400 meters on the treadmill at 7 mph, jump off and do 10 push-ups, then 10 pull-ups, 15 dips, 20 alternating jumping lunges, 30 sit-ups, 15 bicycle abs).

TEENAGE BILLIONAIRE COLLEGE DROPOUTS

Knowledge of STEM (science, technology, engineering, and mathematics), helps anyone especially young teenagers scale their technologies fast. At age 19 Mark Zuckerberg found Facebook in his Harvard University dorm room - becoming the youngest self-made billionaire at age 23.

Elizabeth Holmes founded Theranos at age 19 as a sophomore at Stanford University. Within months, she dropped out of Stanford and became America's youngest self-made female billionaire at age 31 with a $4.5 billion net worth in 2014. Unfortunately, Elizabeth's blood diagnostics company was hit with allegations that its tests were inaccurate causing Forbes to lower her net worth from $4.5 billion in 2014 to $0 in 2016. Per Jina Choi, director of the SEC's San Francisco Regional Office, "The Theranos story is an important lesson for Silicon Valley where innovators who seek to revolutionize and disrupt an industry must tell investors the truth about what their technology can do today, not just what they hope it might do someday."

20s OLYMPIC CHAMPIONS - LEDECKY & MJ

As of 2018, Katie Ledecky is an American swimmer who has won five Olympic gold medals and 14 world championship gold medals - the most in history for a female swimmer.

Michael Jordan, arguably the greatest basketball player of all time, won his first NBA championship at age 28 with the Chicago Bulls. In addition to his 6 NBA championships, he won 5 MVPs, 14 All Star appearances, and 2 Olympic Gold medals - including being on the 1992 Summer Olympic Dream Team with basketball legends Boston Celtics Larry Bird and Los Angeles Lakers Magic Johnson.

20s BUSINESS SENSATIONS - JOBS & BLAKELY

Steve Jobs, one of the greatest inventors of all-time, founded Apple at age 21. Steve brought the world the Macintosh Desktop Computer, the iPod, iTunes, MacBook Pro Laptop, iPhone, MacBook Air, and the iPad.

Unfortunately Steve Jobs died at age 56 from pancreatic cancer. His impact on the world was felt as you can see on YouTube the elaborate funeral held at Apple Headquarters where Al Gore and his favorite band Coldplay came.

Sara Blakely found Spanx at age 27. She kept her day job for two years while working to get Spanx into stores on the side, and quit once Oprah named Spanx as one of her "favorite things." The "Oprah Effect" really works as Sara became the youngest ever self-made female billionaire at age 41.

30s BEST IN TENNIS - FEDERER & SERENA

Tennis is a grueling sport played four times on the world stage annually in Sydney, Paris, London, and New York City.

As of 2018, Roger Federer and Serena Williams are both still winning Tennis Grand Slams in their thirties at an age when athletes go thru "father-time" and "mother-time." Roger's 20 and Serena's 23 Grand Slam singles titles are the most all-time for their respective genders.

30s HUSBAND & WIFE BILLIONAIRES - BEZOS

Jeff Bezos of Amazon was the son of a 16 year old teenage mom and heavy-drinking dad who divorced his mom when Jeff was 17 months old.

Biographer Brad Stone suggests that Bezos' childhood may have contributed to his obsession with success. Two other technology icons, Steve Jobs and Larry Ellison, were also adopted, and the experience is thought by some to have given each a powerful motivation to succeed.

After one year of marriage at age 30, Bezos told his wife MacKenzie that he wanted to quit his job and sell books online. His wife told him to go for it. What a great call as Jeff has changed the world being the richest man in the world with net worth of $145.2 billion as of 2018.

Bezos added that the best way to make the decision to "quit your desk job" is by asking yourself "What does your heart say?" For Bezos, that meant living a life without regrets, especially in old age. Bezos said, "For me, the best way to think about it was to project myself forward to age 80 and say, 'Look, when I'm 80 years old, I want to have minimized the number of regrets that I have.' In most cases, our biggest regrets turn out to be acts of omission. It's paths not taken and they haunt us. We wonder what would have happened. I knew that when I'm 80, I would never regret trying this thing that I was super excited about and it failing. If it failed, fine. I would be very proud of the fact when I'm 80 that I tried. I also knew that it would always haunt me if I didn't try."

In 1982 at age 35, Diane Hendricks was selling custom-built homes and Ken was a roofing contractor. They decided to become life and business partners - getting married and used their lines of credit to secure a loan that enabled them to establish ABC Supply to sell roofing, windows, gutters, and siding for residential and commercial buildings. In 2017, Diane's net worth was $4.3 billion.

40s V-SHAPED CHAMPIONS - THE ROCK

At Age 46, Dwayne Johnson is one of the best athlete to Hollywood success stories being known as "the People's Champion" in wrestling to "the Rock" as an A-list Hollywood actor. In 2017, Forbes named Dwayne the highest paid actor in the world - earning $124 million for the year which was the largest ever recorded on the Forbes celebrity list. Dwyane is known for his chiseled chest and bulging biceps.

As one of the most successful Hollywood actors out there, organizations such as the Los Angeles Lakers bring in Dwayne Johnson to inspire their millionaire young basketball players to not take their playing days for granted because athletes will no longer be elite when their age reaches mid-thirties similar to Dwayne Johnson in wrestling who successful pivoted to acting. Even though Dwayne is wealthy, he stays hungry by reminding himself of all the "hard times" that got him to where he is today. He imagines that his back is against a wall so that the only direction he can go is forward in life. He remembers people doubting him saying he couldn't do this and that but proved everyone wrong. In business, Dwayne always trains his mind to play chess when others are playing checkers in order to win.

At age 41, Dana Torres became the oldest swimmer to compete in the Olympics when she raced at the 2008 Beijing Summer Games. Dana's motto has always been "Age is just a number." Her favorite workout is boxing with the goal to be sore after every workout because she doesn't want anything to be easy.

40s ENTREPRENEURS - SAM WALTON

At age 44, Sam Walton opened the first Walmart in 1962. He named the "Wal" part of company after his family name and "Mart" for supermarket. Never be afraid to name a company that ties in your name such as Sam Walton did because it allows customers to associate the business with you.

Walton had a demanding style, often starting work at 4:30 a.m. Even after becoming a billionaire, Walton continued to drive a pickup truck and wore clothes from his own discount store - Walmart. A married man while launching Walmart, Walton and his wife Helen raised four children, Rob, John, Jim, and Alice. In 1992, Walton wrote in his book "Made in America" that the greatest moment of his life was when President George H. W. Bush (#41) awarded Walton the Presidential Medal of Freedom. Unfortunately, Walton passed away the same year leaving an estimated $100 billion fortune to his wife and four children when he died.

At age 43, Martine Rothblatt moved into biotech after her daughter was diagnosed with pulmonary arterial hypertension. She founded United Therapeutics that sells five FDA-approved pills to help people with the disease. The company is also the world's largest cloner of pigs with a pig 'pharm' in Blacksburg, Virginia. Born as Martin Rothblatt in 1954, Rothblatt would eventually transition into a woman when she came out in 1994. As of year 2018, she has the second highest net worth for transgender women at $390 million ahead of Caitlyn Jenner (Kim Kardashian's parent) and behind Jennifer Pritzker (first person that identifies as transgender to become a billionaire).

50s HOLLYWOOD STARS - TOM CRUISE

At age 56, Tom Cruise is "cruising" thru life after three decades in Hollywood. He's earned every bit of his $570 million net worth having starred and performed most of his dangerous stunts in "Top Gun," Ethan Hunt in "Mission Impossible," and "Jack Reacher." For fitness, Tom enjoys sea-kayaking, fencing, sprinting, lifting weights, and rock-climbing.

Robin Wright now age 52 starred as Claire Underwood in the Netflix political drama "House of Cards," for which she won the Golden Globe Award for Best Actress – Television Series Drama in 2013. Robin is now one of the highest paid actresses in the United States, earning approximately $500,000 per episode for her role in House of Cards.

For fitness, Robin makes 52 look like 32. In preparation for her role in "Wonder Woman" with Gal Gadot, Robin has "warrior-inspired" workouts such as horse riding for an hour, weight training for an hour, and cardio training for an hour. For nutrition during "House of Cards," Robin did the paleo diet that involved avoiding processed food and dairy products. She ate meat, fish, vegetables and fruit. For "Wonder Woman," Robin ate 2,500 calories a day thru raw oats in smoothies with avocado, whole milk and weight-gain powder, three times a day.

50s PURSUE YOUR DREAMS - RAY KROC

At age 52, Ray Kroc drove around USA selling milkshake machines to the owners of drive-in restaurants and struck gold when he met the McDonald's brothers - becoming the largest fast-food business in the world which feeds 1% of the world's population everyday. In the movie "The Founder" and Ray's book "Grinding It Out," Ray's life changed when his CFO Harry Sonneborn steered Ray to the more lucrative direction that "You're not in the hamburger business, you're in the real estate business."

In her mid-50s in 2011, Julie Wainwright launched The RealReal, a second-hand luxury marketplace website. Before the launch, Julie had gone thru the demise of Pets.com and a divorce. After several years, Wainwright realized that her situation personally (divorce) and professionally (company demise) wasn't going to improve unless she took action. Her moment of truth came when she told her girlfriends "I had never created my own business before. I had always been the gun to hire. … But I had to finally say, nobody is going to give me my dream job, so I better figure it out myself." The decision paid off as The RealReal did $10 million sales in first year and $500 million sales in 6 years.

A recent CNBC/SurveyMonkey Small Business Survey of more than 2000 small-business owners found that 30 percent launched a small business between the ages of 55 and 64. And another 22 percent were 65 and older.

60s IS THE NEW 40 - LIAM & ELLEN

Action star Liam Neeson now age 66, makes 66 the new 44. He'll run eight miles a day followed with push-ups and sit ups. Now in his 60s, Liam never skips a warm-up as flexibility is key to longevity and recovery.

Now 60, TV personality Ellen DeGeneres wakes up early for a morning workout of abs and cardio. In 1997, Ellen made waves when she came out as gay on the cover of "Time" and on "The Oprah Winfrey Show," paving the way for many in Hollywood to come out without fear of losing their jobs or public rejection.

60s BUSINESS LAUNCHERS - COL SANDERS

In 1952 at the age of 65, when most people are retiring, Harland

David Sanders began Kentucky Fried Chicken. The world is fortunate that Colonel Harland Sanders did not believe in the adage that "the future belongs to the young" or we would have never tasted the amazing "finger lickin'" fried chicken. Colonel Sanders persevered - handling 1,009 straight rejections before someone agreed to buy his fried chicken recipe.

Laura Ingalls Wilder was 65 years old when "Little House in the Big Woods" was published. Her books are read in America's elementary schools.

70s MOVIE STARS - ARNOLD & MERYL

At age 71, Arnold Schwarzenegger is training for "Terminator 6." Just like the benefits of compound interest when you invest young, Arnold reaped the benefits of exercising young when he began lifting weights at the age of 15. He won the Mr. Universe title at age 20 and went on to win the Mr. Olympia contest seven times. Per Arnold, "70 is only on my passport or my driver's licence, but I feel the same way as I did 20 years ago...I make my movies. I feel useful and productive...I get up at 5am and I ride the bike to the gym. I work out for an hour, then I ride home and have breakfast."

Meryl Streep often deemed the "best actress of her generation" has never gotten plastic surgery. She attributes her life longevity to establishing a work-life balance. After 7pm, Meryl becomes a normal mother and grandmother. She believes that one of the key tips to controlling aging naturally is to control stress, don't overwork yourself, exercise, limit alcohol, and avoid the California sun.

70s POLITICIANS - TRUMP & CLINTON

When you reach your 70s with grand or great-grandchildren, most want to spend time with their family after a life of work, but some want to devote the remaining years of their life in public service leading their country.

In 2016, the United States of America had two candidates in their seventies run to become the 45th President of the United States of America. Donald Trump was the underdog who became the oldest person to ever become President and Hillary Clinton became the first female presidential candidate nominated by a major political party.

80s MOVIE LEGENDS - CLINT EASTWOOD

At age 88, Clint Eastwood stars in his latest film "The Mule" based on the true story of Leo Sharp, a World War II veteran in his 80s, who became a drug dealer and courier for the Sinaloa Cartel.

Eastwood, a lifelong non-smoker, has been conscious of his health and fitness since he was a teenager. From his army experience Clint says "I realized the best way to keep muscles strong, hard, and fit was with weight training." For diet, Clint maintains a low-fat, high protein diet; eats fruits and raw vegetables; takes vitamins, avoids alcohol, and skips sugary drinks. Clint says "Eating healthy food, watching your weight, and exercise should be a lifetime habit - best begun when you are as young as possible."

In 1997 at age 87, Gloria Stuart broke through as a star in her Oscar-nominated performance as "Old Rose" in "Titanic" movie. The secret to Gloria's long life was detailed in her memoir "I Just Kept Hoping" where she considered "Titanic" her last chance to finally prove she could be a first-rank actress. Research published in Psychological Science found that people who report having a strong purpose in life tend to outlive their peers.

80s AMERICAN SAGES - GINSBURG & BUFFETT

At age 85, two-time cancer survivor Ruth Bader Ginsburg is the oldest justice on the Supreme Court who was appointed by President Bill Clinton in 1993. When asked about the most important person in her life after losing her husband in 2010 and her best friend Justice Scalia in 2016, Ruth responded "My personal trainer." Justice Ginsburg's workouts last 90-minutes where she warms up for five-minutes on an elliptical machine followed by light stretching. Then comes strength training - performing 3x10 sets for the machine bench chest press, leg curls, leg presses, chest flies and lat pull-downs while stretching the muscle groups being exercised in between sets. For balance, Justice Ginsburg performs one-legged squats. Next up is 10 pushups followed by a 30 second plank hold and then 30 second side plank holds. To promote leg strength and hip flexibility, she does step ups to knee raise on an 18 inch high box. Finally to ensure Justice Ginsburg can use a toilet unassisted, she sits on a bench holding a medicine ball and tosses the ball to her trainer while standing up and sitting back down after catching the ball.

At age 88, legendary investor Warren Buffett is widely praised for his adherence to value investing and his personal frugality despite his immense wealth. Once a year, Warren invites students from the top business schools including Harvard Business School, Northwestern Kellogg School of Management, and Vanderbilt Owen Graduate School of Management to Berkshire Hathaway's headquarters in Omaha, Nebraska. In 2016, I was fortunate to have been selected to meet Warren at his annual MBA event. My favorite quote from Warren on success was "In the world of business, the people who are most successful are those who are doing what they love... Think about it. ... Doing what we love is a major contributor to our happiness as humans. And, more important, knowing what you love should be a top priority."

Personally, if you're feeling less excited about life than Warren, Warren suggests you imagine the people in your life as publicly traded companies - some will succeed where their value will rise while some will flounder where their value fall. In one hour, you have to pick one of your classmates to own 10 percent of for the rest of your life. As you write that person's name down, list the reasons or qualities that caused you to pick that person. Next, think about someone who you would "sell short" which means you expect their value to decrease. Consider the behaviors of the two people you picked and make a list. On one side, you list the qualities of the person who you want to own 10 percent of, and on the other side you list the qualities of the person who you want to short 10 percent of. Per Warren, "When it comes to the person you expect to succeed, you will find that these are not things you are born with, like the ability to kick a football or sing a high C, they are qualities that you actually generate for yourself like generosity, humor, forgiveness. Work on developing the personality of people you admire, while ridding yourself of the qualities you dislike in others."

Professionally, Warren has a three-step rule of focus for success.
1. Write down a list of your top 25 career goals.
2. Circle the five most important goals that truly speak to you.
3. Eliminate the other 20 goals you listed. Warren says "these 20 goals are not urgent priorities. You should put all your effort and focus into achieving your top five most important goals. The rest are merely distractions that will get in the way of you reaching your ultimate success."

90s HOLLYWOOD LEGENDS - BETTY & STAN

At age 96, Betty White was honored at the 2018 Emmy Awards for 80 years in Hollywood. Betty is a pioneer of television - being the first woman to produce a sitcom (Life with Elizabeth).

Researchers who study longevity analyse the traits and habits followed by centenarians (people who live until age 100) in places such as Okinawa, Japan, the Nicoya Peninsula in Costa Rica and Loma Linda in California, all known as "blue zones" where the number of old people living there are high. Old people in these "blue zones" drink moderately, don't stress, stay social, and remain active.

Betty exhibits these traits as she stays active, works for good causes, and stays positive. She claims her life longevity is due to her sense of humor and optimism. Betty says "I know it sounds corny, but I try to see the funny side and the upside, not the downside. I get bored with people who complain about this or that, it's such a waste of time. It sounds so trite, but a lot of people will pick out something to complain about, rather than say 'Hey, that was great!' It's not hard to find great stuff if you look."

Stan Lee lived until age 95. He was the Marvel Comics' primary creative leader for two decades creating popular fictional superheroes including Spider-Man, the X-Men, Iron Man, Thor, the Hulk, the Fantastic Four, Black Panther, Daredevil, Doctor Strange, Scarlet Witch and Ant-Man.

Personally, Stan lived long due to finding the perfect love partner as he remained married with his wife for 70 years until her passing one year before his. Stan's advice is "Just pick the right girl."

Professionally, Stan says the reason he continues working even after age 90 is "That I'm happiest when I'm working. If I'm not working, I feel like I'm wasting my time. Most people say "I can't wait to retire so I can play golf"...Playing golf, you get together with your friends for an afternoon - talk and have fun...I do that in the office and we're accomplishing more than hitting a ball into a hole."

Regarding death, Stan says "It's just something you have to accept, because there isn't a damn thing you can do to stop it. I guess I'll keep working till I drop. You know how the cowboys die with their boots on? I guess I'm going to die at the keyboard of a computer."

90s POLITICAL ROYALTY - GHWB & QEII

Until his death at age 94, George H.W. Bush lived an amazing life. George served as the 41st President of the United States from 1989 to 1993. When he turned 90, he was still a daredevil - skydiving near his Kennebunkport, Maine Summer home.

In 2018, never before has one President eulogized another President who was also his father. George W. Bush loved his father. In his last phone call, George W. asked his ailing father whether he wanted to go to the hospital. The former President answered no and said that he was ready to be with Barbara - his wife of 73 years, and their late daughter Robin who died of leukemia as a child. During George H.W. Bush's eulogy in Washington D.C.,

George W. Bush cried when he finished his last line about his father saying "George H.W. Bush was the best father a son or daughter could have."

At age 92, Queen Elizabeth II is healthy and strong. She loves being around her horses and dogs and keeping up with them helps the Queen stay fit. Regarding nutrition the Queen "eats to live rather than living to eat." Her Chef McGrady says "Many people will do anything it takes to get an extra piece of cake or will revolve their life around food. Food is meant to fuel you in your day, not your day to be focused on food." She enjoys a cup of Earl Grey tea (without milk or sugar) in the morning along with a bowl of Special K cereal. For lunch, she eats fish and veggies. And the Queen finishes the day with a dinner meal of either lamb, roast beef, or salmon.

LIVING PAST 100 - ROBERTA MCCAIN

Congratulations if you are over the age of 100. In 2010, 82.8 percent of centenarians were female as most males die on average three years earlier than woman born on the same day.

Factors such as smoking, drinking, overeating, and lack of exercise may partly explain why the gender gap varies so widely between males and females living until age 100. For instance, Russian men die 13 years earlier than Russian women because they drink vodka and smoke more heavily.

Here are examples of notable people who lived past age 100.

Queen Elizabeth known as "The Queen Mother" lived until age 101. She was the wife of King George VI and mother of Queen Elizabeth II who is now 92 years old. Dr. Michael Gordon, the program director of palliative care at Baycrest Geriatric Health Care System, met the Queen Mother and says "Even being in your 80s is no big deal. We accelerate the aging process if we smoke, drink heavily, eat poorly, don't exercise, and are overstressed. Successful aging is measured both in quantity of years and quality of life - retaining enough enthusiasm and vitality to make life worth living."

Albert Hofmann, the Swiss chemist who discovered and uses the psychedelic drug LSD, lived until age 102. He remained active touring the world for lectures and stayed active. During a 2006 LSD symposium in Switzerland, Albert revealed that his secret to long life had nothing to do with drugs. LSD's most famous user is Apple CEO Steve Jobs who often asked potential Apple employees during interviews how many times they had dropped acid. At age 101, Albert formally sent the following letter to Steve Jobs but never received a reply "I understand from media accounts that you feel LSD helped you creatively in your development of Apple Computers and your personal spiritual quest." Albert mentions that he ate two eggs with his muesli for breakfast every morning.

Roberta McCain now age 106 is the mother of U.S. Senator and former POW John McCain. She had to experience the heartbreaking experience of burying her son who died in 2018 of brain cancer at the age of 81. John McCain wrote a book that detailed his mother's life longevity stating "My mother was raised to be a strong, determined woman who thoroughly enjoyed life, and always tried to make the most of her opportunities. I am grateful to her for the strengths she taught me, even if I have not possessed them as well and as comfortably as she does. She has an endless curiosity about the world, about natural history and, even more so, human history."

CHAPTER 19

SUPERCENTENARIAN FITNESS SECRETS

Keep away from people who try to belittle your ambition. Small people always do that, but the really great make you feel that you too, can become great

- Mark Twain

200 SUPERCENTENARIANS WORLDWIDE

A supercentenarian is someone who has lived to or passed their 110th birthday. We all want to age gracefully and enjoy time in resort communities as described in Jimmy Buffett's famous "Margaritaville" song.

Over 1,500 supercentenarians have been documented in history. Jeanne Calment of France, who died in 1997 at age 122 years 164 days, had the longest documented human lifespan. The oldest man ever verified is Jiroemon Kimura of Japan who died in 2013 at age 116 years 54 days. Supercentenarians are extremely rare individuals. There are likely 60 in the United States and 200-300 world wide.

Research has found that supercentenarians remain free of major age-related diseases (e.g. stroke, cardiovascular disease, dementia, cancer, Parkinson's disease, and diabetes) until the very end of life when they die of exhaustion of organ reserve which is the ability to return organ function to homeostasis.

Professor Nobuyoshi Hirose of Keio University, geneticist George Church of Harvard Medical School, Thomas Perls of Boston University's New England Centenarian Study, and Robert D. Young of UCLA's Gerontology Research Group are all devoted to research reversing aging. Each have enrolled supercentenarians and their children for study. With 200-300 living supercentenarians, Thomas Perls has enrolled more than 60 supercentenarians which is the most in the world. Their research suggests that approximately 30% of human longevity is hardwired in our DNA and 70% is due to our lifestyle and environment. Thomas believes it would take 500 to 1000 genomes to truly unlock their secrets.

In addition to research labs, a number of Silicon Valley billionaires have funnelled their own millions into the anti-ageing cause with PayPal's Peter Thiel investing in Breakout Labs to tackle degenerative diseases, Google's Larry Page allocating $750 million of company dollars into Calico for biotech research, and J. Craig Venture's Human Longevity doing genome sequencing. Larry Ellison, Sergey Brin, Paul F. Glenn, and Dmitry Itskov are also funding research into longevity science.

With Jeanne Calment holding the record for oldest person to ever live at 122.5 years old, Moldovan businessman Dmitry Kaminskiy pledges a $1 million prize to the first person who can live to be 123 years old. He hopes this million dollar gift will trigger a new group of "supercentenarians."

LAND OF IMMORTALS - HARA HACHI BU

Japan currently has the greatest number of known centenarians of any nation in the world with 69,785 older than age 100 of which 88 percent are women. Each year, Japan celebrates the lives of its centenarians with a public holiday known as the "Respect for the Aged Day" when those over age 100 receive a letter of congratulations and a commemorative sake cup from Prime Minister Shinzo Abe. When Japanese people have to visit the hospital, they don't worry about cost as Japan's health care system is one of the most accessible in the world where the government pays 70 percent of the cost of all health procedures.

Okinawa, Japan where hundreds of residents are over 100 years old, adopt the "Okinawa Diet" eating three servings of fish a week, wholegrains, vegetables, tofu, kombu seaweed, squid, and octopus - which are rich in taurine that lower cholesterol and blood pressure.

Okinawans adopt an eating habit called 'hara hachi bu' – where people eat until they're 80% full. This habit is based on the delay between the stomach becoming full and the brain receiving this signal, which experts agree takes 20 minutes – so many of us who eat too quickly during this "delay" period end up having eaten more than we should have.

SUPERCENTENARIAN - LIVING PAST AGE 110

Supercentenarians lived past age 110 by exhibiting the below habits. Start incorporating these into your life to live longer and happier. Professor

Vladimir Khavinson, the past President of the European region of the International Association of Gerontology and Geriatrics says "A clean environment, fresh food, physical activity and medical advances can allow people who are young today to live until age 120."

Purpose: Maude Harris lived until age 111 says "I think I have lived so long because I was interested in this world. God put us here for a purpose. It was not to improve our own self, but to make a world that is fair and livable for everyone. We need to have more tolerance for different opinions and treat others with respect."

Independence: Besse Cooper who lived to age 116 loved to do things herself such as chopping down her own Christmas tree when she was age 86.

Exercise: Rose M Theissen who lived to age 110 made fitness a habit as she started exercising and weight lifting in her 30's. Being married to a pharmacist, vitamins were also important. Exercise is great for maintaining a healthy weight and decreasing your risk of heart disease.

Dancing: Ethel Lang who lived until age 114 loved to dance. She also never smoked or drank alcohol.

Love: Henry Allingham who lived until age 113 says "Whisky and wild women helped me live long happily!"

Laugh: still both alive at age 110, Britain's Alf Smith and Robert Weighton credit their old age to having a great sense of humor. Robert says "I think laughter is extremely important. Most of the trouble in the world is caused by people taking themselves too seriously."

Sing: Christian Mortensen who lived until age 115 credits his long happy life to singing, keeping a positive attitude, staying away from alcohol, drinking lots of water, and having great friends. Singing involves deep breathing - good for the nervous system.

Faith: Bernando LaPallo who lived until age 114 took his father's advice who lived until age 98 to "have faith in God and he'll take care of you."

Alcohol Abstinence: Alexander Imich who lived to age 111 stayed healthy by abstaining from alcohol.

Smoking Cessation: Susannah Mushatt who lived until age 116 didn't smoke or drink.

Nutrition: Chiyo Miyako who lived until age 117 was the oldest person in the world. She ate heart-healthy fish, tofu, seaweed, and octopus - all of which carry a low risk for some cancers and arteriosclerosis.

Morning Eggs: Emma Morano who lived until age 117 ate 3 eggs for breakfast everyday.

Chocolate: Jeanne Calment who lived until age 122 is the oldest person to ever live. She credits her youthful appearance to eating 2 pounds of chocolate a week.

No Junk Food: Besse Cooper who lived until age 116 said her secret to longevity was from avoiding junk food and "minding her own business."

Sleep: Misao Okawa who lived until age 117 slept eight hours a night.

Kindness: Gertrude Weaver who lived to age 116 advises aspiring supercentenarians the values of being kind to others and treating them as you would wish to be treated.

Positivity: Holocaust survivor Alice Herz-Sommer who lived until age 111 says a long happy life is all about being positive.

Calm: Sarah Knauss-Clark who lived until age 119 says the reason for her longevity stemmed from her tranquil personality where she never gets fazed - even the worst of news.

No swearing: Benjamin Holcomb who lives until age 111 was a happy man who never said negative things about anyone. He never drank alcohol, never smoked, and never cursed.

Brainwork: Anna Stoehr who lived until age 114 kept her mind busy by playing scrabble, cooking, cleaning, and socializing with friends.

4:44AM WORKOUTS TO AGE 200

As a martial artist and power athlete, my mission is to inspire the world to make fitness a habit to live past age 120. Now 30 years young and married, people think I'm not old enough to drink - assuming I'm under 21.

Living in Boston, I stay connected with Vanderbilt University. When I come to freshman summer send-off events, the Vanderbilt admissions director as well as incoming Freshman all thought I was an incoming 18 year old Freshman! I took it as a compliment letting them know I'm old enough to be their uncle - having completed my MBA, married, and boosted people's confidence thru JustHuynh Fitness. To give back, I share advice with students and alumni on how to stay healthy and young.

As you age, you should incorporate warming up and cooling down into your workout routine to avoid injury.

BULLETPROOF WARMUP - INJURY FREE

Your body is like a car that needs care to minimize maintenance from injuries. Just like in cold weather when you should warm-up your car to avoid a breakdown, your body needs a warm-up before exercising.

Here is the bulletproof exercise warm-up routine, with approximate time for each exercise, that JustHuynh Fitness teaches all of our members.
- 30 Jumping Jax (30 seconds)
- 10 Each Jumping Alternate Forward Lunges (1 minute)
- 10 Each Alternate High Knees (30 seconds)
- 10 Each Butt Kicks (30 seconds)
- Side Lunge 15 second each side and 15 second down middle (1 minute)
- Cross-over Toe Touch: 15 second each side (30 seconds)
- Quad Hold: 15 second each side (30 seconds)
- Pretzel Stretch: 30 second hold (1 minute)
- Hurdle Stretch: 30 second each side (1 minute)
- Glute Stretch: 30 second each side (1 minute)
- Leg Cycle: 30 second forward and reverse circles (1 minute)
- Lying Leg Crossover 15 sec each side (30 seconds)
- Standing Wall Calf Stretch: 15 second each side Twice (1 minute)
- Leg side swings: 20 each (1 minute)
- Forward leg swings: 20 each (1 minute)

POST WORKOUT RECOVERY - CATABOLISM

Muscle growth begins the moment you stop lifting or performing high intensity exercises, and that growth can't happen without a proper recovery protocol. When you lift heavy or partake in high intensity training, muscles suffer microtears and are actually broken down via a process called catabolism. If you want to get the most from every workout, you need to prioritize post-workout recovery. Follow these tips that we teach our JustHuynh Fitness members to maximize recovery and be in tip-top shape.

Post workout protein: After a great workout, remember to consume a post-workout protein, such as Whey, to feed the muscles for growth like Hugh Jackman's Wolverine mutant-healing ability.

Schedule ample recovery time between workouts: While many people recommend two days of rest between workouts involving the same muscle group, there's no one-size-fits-all solution for recovery time. Factors like age and fitness level influence how much rest we need. If you notice performance decreasing between workouts for particular muscle groups, rest more.

Massage: get a massage from a therapist or self-massage with foam rollers, massage sticks and even baseballs or tennis balls to reduce muscle tightness and improve range of motion. Massaging before a workout can help you loosen up to improve muscle function. Foam rolling after a workout can help flush out toxins and lactic acid from a muscle.

Focus On Quality Sleep: At least seven hours of sleep is ideal. For focus, set a "technology blackout" on TV and phones after a certain time like 9 p.m. Research suggests taking a 30 minute nap two hours after a workout as sleep helps your heart, blood pressure, stress levels and weight management. Take advantage of that nap pod at work or take a team timeout at the desk.

Hydrate: Drink lots of water as dehydration can reduce your performance and delay recovery. Experts suggest a minimum daily water intake for males at 3.7 liters (15 cups) and 2.7 liters (11 cups) for females.

Cut alcohol: Research suggests more than two alcoholic drinks can reduce the body's ability to recover. The empty calories from alcohol also lead to weight gain.

Ice Bath: After a tough workout session, practice, or game, many athletes use ice baths or ice cups on their body to bring down inflammation and speed up recovery. Submerge your body in the cold water or ice cup for 10 minutes and repeat this as needed.

Steam Room and Sauna: The heat from a sauna increases the body's circulation which removes metabolic waste products like hydrogen ions, while carrying oxygen and other nutrients necessary to help repair tissue used during the workout - helping you avoid or recover from muscle and joint ache. The sauna triggers heat shock proteins that push the body into optimal repair and rebuild mode. Saunas also helps you sleep more soundly. Using the steam room increases blood flow and circulation, relaxes stiff joints and muscles, helps reduce stress, deep cleanses the skin, helps eliminate toxins, and relieves congestion of upper respiratory mucous membranes if you're dealing with a cough. The steam rooms also causes you to sweat thus helps you lose water weight.

CHAPTER 20

TIME WASTERS

If I had eight hours to chop down a tree, I'd spend six sharpening my ax

- Abraham Lincoln

TIME WASTED PER DAY - 6 HOURS

People are chronic procrastinators where we tend to delay finishing tasks by browsing mindlessly on forms of media called "visual crack" from our laptops, phones, tv, or games. The rise of technology has enhanced life, but has also taken away your precious time on non-value add activities.

In one of social media guru Gary Vaynerchuk's speaking engagements, Gary asked the crowd "How many people waste 10 hours a day of their life?" 10% of people raise their hands. When Gary asked "How many people waste 6 hours a day?" then 80% of people raised their hands. That's 42 hours a week which is the equivalent of a working week!

Time is money and Gary wants you to put a value on your time to reduce pursuing time-wasting activities. Ask yourself "How much is your time worth?" If you're making $50 an hour, then by wasting 42 hours a week that is $2,000 a week's worth of time you're wasting or over $100,000 in time value wasted for the year. Over a span of 40 years, that is $4 million worth of time wasted. Think about what you could do with $4 million? Hopefully this motivates you to make better use of your time for your physical, mental, and financial wellness.

SOCIAL MEDIA ADDICTION - DOPAMINE

Remember you only need to exercise a minimum 3 hours a week to meet the World Health Organization's health guideline - ensuring a balance of cardio and strength training. Only 23% of people worldwide meet this.

Time Waster: An alarming 2 hours a day are spent on social media as people kill time by scrolling to see their friends, frenemies, or celebrities - often times getting depressed as they are not having as much joy compared to their friends. Salesforce CEO Marc Benioff has even suggested a social media tax similar to that for cigarettes.

Dopamine: Social media apps provide people with short-term dopamine hits thru likes, comments, and views. If you haven't yet realized, the phone is a "slot machine" that exploits your vulnerability psychologically for your addiction in social media's "Attention Economy."

Social Media Purge: As you enter different phases of your life, there will be friends who you need to eliminate from taking your precious time. To focus, I purged my Facebook and Linkedin by eliminating 1,000 connections from each platform who did not contribute positively to my personal and professional life. The process took time and was painful but got easier as I clicked delete because the simple question I asked was "Can I call this person right this second and have a great conversation where we each cared about each other?" If no, then I deleted them. With time as the most precious resource, purging unneeded connections will free up time to pursue your goals without haters or negative people being in your way.

WEBSITE ADDICTION - BROWSER BLOCKER

People have many go-to websites for sports, fashion, and world news - thus wasting time that could have spent on exercise or a productive task.

Website Blockers: website browsers now allow you to enter websites to block that will help you dedicate time for exercise and life productivity.

GAMING DISORDER - HIKIKOMORI

Video games are a time killer with the World Health Organization labelling "gaming" as a health disorder. With the rise of digital connections and elimination of physical interaction, many people are now more socially awkward - suffering a problem called "Hikikomori" which is the complete social withdrawal from real life into a virtual life. Gamers miss out on the beauty of nature, loving relationships and satisfaction of contributing to a better world, all for a fake life. If this sounds like you, cut down your gaming to get out and meet people who could be positive additions in your life.

ONLINE TV ADDICTION - BLOOD CLOTS & VTE

As of year 2018, you need to stop binge watching as 70% of online streaming subscribers watch 5 shows a day like it's their part time job. You can learn and laugh thru TV, but 35 hours of TV a week is overkill. Instead, cut back on TV to ensure you're getting 3 hours of exercise each week. A 2015 study by the University of Minnesota revealed that people who binge-watch TV are likely to develop fatal blood clots in their legs.

VTE: Prolonged TV watching can increase the likelihood of developing Venous thromboembolism (VTE) because it's harder for blood to return to other parts of the body due to continued sitting. VTE can travel through veins and lodge in the lungs, which can cause serious health complications. Per the Centers for Disease Control and Prevention, 60,000 to 100,000 Americans die from VTE annually.

TIME WASTED AT WORK - 2 HOURS

On the job, the average worker wastes 2 hours a day. According to a survey conducted by Sugarcookie, 59% of people waste company money watching porn on the job. In addition to porn, employees waste time online shopping, scheduling their online date, or playing mindless app games.

SAVE 1 HOUR A DAY

As mentioned, the World Health Organization's guideline is 3 hours of exercise a week. Just cutting "1 hour" of your wasted time for 3 days each week can be used to perform cardio such as martial arts and power athletics with JustHuynh Fitness. More optimal is saving an additional 3 hours for weight lifting. This allows you to stay HEALTHY and PRODUCTIVE - no longer needing to pay the price of inactivity.

CHAPTER 21

EAT TO LIVE

It is health that is real wealth and not pieces of gold and silver

- Mahatma Gandhi

EATING APPROACH - 6 SMALL MEALS

Remember every 3,500 calories that you reduce is equivalent to 1 pound which can be done by cutting back 500 calories a day. Many people "Live to Eat" consuming thousands of calories every meal. The best way to stay disciplined is "Eat to Live" where you view food as the gas for your body to function just like a car. Be conscious of the saying "Once on the lips, forever on the hips!" meaning any unhealthy food you eat will get stored on your body that could lead to serious health issues.

As an active person thru exercise, you'll be burning calories throughout the day so plan 6 small meals throughout the day such as eating at 8AM, 10AM, 12PM, 3PM, 6PM, and 8PM.

The three key macronutrients are protein, fat, and carbohydrates. Carbs and protein have 4 calories per gram. Fat is 9 calories per gram. Protein builds muscle. Fat is stored energy in brain, nerves, hair, skin, and nails. Carbs are fuel for exercise. Eat complex carbs like whole grains, beans, fruits, and veggies. Stop eating simple carbs from candy, cookies, fruit juice, and soda.

Protein maintains muscle and makes you feel more full. There are a variety of options ranging from fish, skinless poultry like chicken, low fat dairy, eggs, and tofu. Good sources of fat for the heart are olive and canola oil, peanut butter, and avocado. Avoid saturated fat animal sources like beef, pork, and lamb which increase risk of heart attack and stroke. In terms of vegetables, you can choose from lettuce, cucumbers, tomatoes, and spinach. To stay full, you can consumer 35g of fiber a day as fiber doesn't affect calories since it can't be digested.

GROCERY LIST

Once you establish your 3 main meals and 3 surrounding snack meals that hit your calorie count, make a shopping list and stick to that list because you will eat whatever is in your refrigerator. Consuming homemade meals are the best as you know what you're putting into your body as opposed to the mystery in calorie and macronutrients in dine-out meals.

POTATO CHIP MARKETING VICTIMS

In line with your healthy grocery shopping habits, you have to be extremely careful of "potato chip" marketing tactics when you're shopping in-store or ads seen online.

Packaged food companies study consumer psychology to profit from "potato chip marketing" where more than 90% of product sales come from less than 10% of the customers with target weight more than 200 pounds. The company's goal is for the overweight customers to consume twice the amount per serving as a normal weight person. At times, marketing executives refuse to attend their own focus groups as they don't want to view their future victims in person and prefer to review transcripts in their cushy offices. They might report to their family over dinner "If my team can get each of 200 pound women up to 210 pounds in a month by eating our potato chips, we'll make our second-quarter sales numbers and I'll get the bonus we need to take a vacation in Paris." The most ironic part of junk-food executives is that the enthusiastic promoters (marketing executives) personally avoid the very products they are pushing to their target 200 pound customers.

EATING OUT - HIPPOCRATES HEALTH

Dining out at restaurants or events and especially while travelling is dangerous as the portions are typically big and unhealthy. As such, ask for the menu ahead of time so you can pick healthy options and ask the chef to split the meal into portions so you can take home leftovers instead of trying to finish the whole meal there. Keep in mind Hippocrates quote "If we could give every individual the right amount of nourishment and exercise, not too little and not too much, we would have the safest way to health."

COFFEE, COCONUT, TEA, BONE BROTH

Regarding coffee, you can save on average $7,800 a year by going with water instead of consuming 3 cups of coffee a day for 5 times each week at $10 per drink. According to Food Standards Australia New Zealand, a regular flat white (similar to a small latte or cappuccino) could have as much as 282mg of caffeine in one serving. More than 400mg of caffeine per day can put you at risk of increased heart rate, heartburn, jittering, anxiety, muscle spasms, stomach cramps, insomnia, and headaches. Watch the daily caffeine.

Healthier drinks are coconut water, tea, and bone broth. Coconut water contains natural electrolytes that make for a great post-workout drink, without added sugar and artificial sweeteners found in sports drinks, to help replenish fluids lost during exercise.

Japanese who live in Okinawa Japan, known as the "Land of the Immortals," drink 6 cups of green tea a day for the bioactive compounds that improve health. Green tea contains large amounts of a catechin, natural antioxidants, called EGCG that help prevent cell damage, heart disease, type 2 diabetes, cancer, weight gain, Alzheimer's and Parkinson's.

Cooking bones from meat, poultry or fish for an extended period of time releases nutrients from the marrow within the bones and connective tissues. The main nutrient, collagen, helps with muscle and bone health to reduce signs of aging. For Vietnamese, we consume bone broth in pho.

ALCOHOL - PANCREATITIS & ASIAN GLOW

Inventor Thomas Edison once said "I have better use for my brain than to poison it with alcohol. To put alcohol in the human brain is like putting sand in the bearings of an engine." Drinking is a popular stress reliever from the weekly job grind, but you can celebrate in others ways such as thru group exercise and sober free gatherings to avoid inflammation of the pancreas that could lead to a burst appendix requiring gallbladder removal - such as DJ Avicii experienced before committing suicide.

Drinking tends to bring out a dark side in people. I've attended company holiday parties where an employee got intoxicated than punched their boss in front of 1,000 co-workers. When drinking around family or friends, some people say hurtful things which ruins relationships. On a nutritional front, alcohol provides no nutritional value to your body.

Philip J. Brooks, an investigator with the Division of Metabolism and Health Effects at the National Institute on Alcohol Abuse and Alcoholism, cites that 33% of East Asians suffer from "alcohol red flush reaction" which is an enzyme deficiency that increases risk of esophageal cancer. Alcohol is metabolised primarily thru enzymes in the liver via two major steps: conversion of alcohol to acetaldehyde and then to acetate. 40% of East Asians lack one of the enzymes needed to convert acetaldehyde to acetate which is serious as acetaldehyde is classified as a 'probable human carcinogen' by the US Environmental Protection Agency. The best way to curb this risk is to reduce or stop alcohol consumption.

SMOKING & KING JAMES I

Per the Centers for Disease Control and Prevention in 2018, 15.5% of Americans or 37.8 million adults smoked. King James I of England once said "Smoking is a custom loathsome to the eye, hateful to the nose, harmful to the brain, and dangerous to the lungs." Cigarette smoking is the leading cause of preventable death accounting for 480,000 deaths each year.

WEED CBD PAIN MANAGEMENT

Weed is a growing industry that employs 200,000 in the United States - generating $11 billion in sales with projections of $75 billion in year 2030. The two forms of marijuana are THC which produces a "high" and CBD which doesn't give a "high." CBD is commonly used for therapeutic benefits such as pain management.

Per Harvard physician Jordan Tishler, "You should not use cannabis for peak performance, but cannabis is good for pain control after your workout." When you take CBD, you will have impaired performance, decreased reaction time, and poor hand-eye coordination, which is why you should never take CBD during a workout. Olympians, UFC fighters, NBA basketball, and NFL athletes all agree with the "pain management" benefits of CBD. After fighting Conor McGregor, UFC fighter Nate Diaz smoked vaped CBD oil during his press conference saying "CBD helps with the healing process and inflammation so you want to get these after fights." In 2018, the World Anti-Doping Agency, which governs drug testing for the Olympics and UFC, removed CBD from its list of banned substances because the agency is convinced by CBD's therapeutic properties. In the NFL, Martellus Bennett says "89% of player use CBD because you don't want to be popping pills as those pills will eat at your liver and kidneys." In the NBA, Kenyon Martin says 85% use CBD for similar reasons.

In 2018, Massachusetts opened its first two recreational dispensaries (Cultivate in Leicester and NETA in Northampton) that combined for $2.6 million sales in their first week. It's a win-win situation for medical patients as medical marijuana is legal and a win for the State of Massachusetts as recreational marijuana is projected (assuming 15% of adults use marijuana) to bring in $61.9 million of taxes for 2019 and $154.2 million for 2020 - at a 20% tax rate. This is a law enforcement win as well with marijuana advocate Nevada State Senator Tick Segerblom saying "cops don't have to waste their time arresting marijuana users now that it is legal - 588,000 Americans were arrested in 2016 for marijuana possession." Following Denver's success with 300 recreational stores where there has been no increase in neighborhood crime or loitering, Boston Mayor Martin Walsh hopes "the human toll is worth the tax" and U.S. House of Representative from MA Joe Kennedy says "legalization is our best chance to ensure that addiction is treated as a public health issue - not a criminal justice one."

In terms of costs, the average customer will purchase an eighth (3.5 grams or ⅛ of an ounce) of weed for $60 - purchasing 1.6 ounces per month for a total average spend of $768 a month. When purchasing CBD at stores, look for 8:1 and 4:1 CBD:THC ratios for optimal pain management. CBD experts recommend taking 1-6 mg of CBD for every 10 pounds you weigh so 15 mg - 90 mg for a 150 pound person.

If you follow JustHuynh Fitness' bulletproof warm-up, cardio and strength training, and post-recovery tips, you should be able to recover on your own without CBD. However, if you do need CBD, try your best to not have to depend on it as much.

OPIOIDS - U.S. CONSUMES 80% WORLD SUPPLY

In 2017, the Trump Administration declared the opioid crisis as a public health emergency. Per the CDC, more than 140 Americans die every day or 62,000 annually die from an opioid overdose.

Opioid medications otherwise known as pain relievers, are the most widely prescribed class of drugs worldwide. Even though the United States represents about five percent of the world's population, it consumes 80 percent of the global opioid supply. That is astounding.

Scientifically in the brain, "liking" and "wanting" are two different psychological experiences. "Liking" refers to the delight one might experience EATING a chocolate cookie. "Wanting" is our desire when we EYE the plate of cookies on the table during a meeting. Dopamine is responsible for "wanting" – not for "liking."

All drugs of abuse such as opioids or heroin trigger a surge of dopamine – a rush of "wanting" – in the brain that makes you crave more drugs. With repeated drug use, the "wanting" grows, while your "liking" of the drug stagnates or even decreases - known as tolerance.

Most people begin taking prescription opioids not for pleasure but rather from a need to manage their pain, often on the recommendation of a doctor. When people use specific drugs over time, the brain requires higher and higher levels of dopamine to feel the pleasure it once felt naturally.

Harvard University performed an analysis in 2014 and 2015 that revealed opioid manufacturers paid hundreds of doctors across America six-figure sums for speaking, consulting and other services. Thousands of other doctors were paid over $25,000 during that time. During those two years, 811,000 doctors wrote prescriptions to Medicare patients with half writing at least one prescription for opioids. Shockingly, 54% of those doctors or 200,000 physicians -- received a payment from pharmaceutical companies that make opioids.

In 2001 Purdue Pharma spent $200 million on aggressive marketing strategies to promote the addictive OxyContin drug and targeted doctors across the country with campaigns that misrepresented safety of its product.

To stop the aggressive marketing of dangerous addictive drugs, the Trump Administration has vowed to launch ad campaigns so young people can see "the devastation and ruination drugs cause people and people's lives."

Drug addiction typically gets people's attention when a celebrity dies - singer Tom Petty, actress Carrie Fisher, singer Prince, actor Philip Seymour Hoffman, actor Heath Ledger, singer Cory Monteith, comedian Chris Farley, HQ Trivia CEO Colin Kroll, and many more.

Exercise can kill addiction. In 2007, Eminem was 230 pounds as his painkiller addiction caused him to eat tons of food. Eminem mentioned the stomachaches were from the coating on the Vicodin and the Valium. When Eminem got out of rehab, he faced the difficulty of satisfying the "addict's brain" as he couldn't sleep when he was off the drugs so he turned to exercise which gave him a natural endorphin high and helped him sleep. Eminem is just one of many examples where exercise can help withdrawal to overcome drug addiction. By adopting exercise as a new habit, you'll reduce stress, anxiety, and depression - the major symptoms of withdrawal.

CHAPTER 22

Love & Sex

Love alone will not bring happiness in marriage, nor will sex alone. But when these two beautiful emotions are blended, marriage may bring about a state of mind which is closest to the spiritual that one may ever know during earthly existence

- Napoleon Hill

MALE ERECTILE DYSFUNCTION

There are personal topics that men keep to themselves such as skin care, hair loss, erectile dysfunction (ED) and premature ejaculation. We see evidence of this stigma in the TV Show "Office US," where Andy gets defensive about his erectile dysfunction when co-workers asked if he had "penile softiosis." Erectile dysfunction is the inability for men to maintain an erection sufficient for sex - affecting 30 million American men according to the James Buchanan Brady Urological Institute at Johns Hopkins University. The Massachusetts Male Aging Study reported that 40% of men are affected with ED at age 40 and nearly 70% of men are affected with ED at age 70.

Psychologically, ED can be caused by poor communication with your sex partner, stress, anxiety, depression, and fatigue. Physically, ED can be caused by smoking, drug abuse (cocaine, marijuana, heroin), spinal cord injury, heart disease, diabetes, obesity, low testosterone, high cholesterol, high blood pressure (hypertension), sleep disorders, alcohol, and insufficient exercise (i.e. 180 minutes of exercise per week for adults).

What's dangerous is that having ED is a precursor of future underlying health conditions such as heart attack, strokes, high cholesterol, diabetes, hypertension, depression, sleep disorders, or hormonal imbalances.

In order for men to satisfy their love partner, some spend money on medications that relax muscles and boost blood flow to the penis for an easier erection. These medications typically last for 2 hours with some side effects such as headache, indigestion, nasal congestion, and impaired vision.

Infertility is also a major issue. Influenced by bodybuilders to get "huge," many men take steroids as a teenager and pay the price when they want to give birth with their wife in their thirties because steroids shut down your body's natural production of testosterone. Millions of sperm are released during sex and men who suffer infertility feel dejected when their semen analysis reveals a zero sperm count - thus preventing the men from getting his wife pregnant to give birth. This is shocking to many men who deem themselves macho because they work out, have tattoos, and have muscles, but their biggest mistake is taking steroids. A 2017 infertility survey conducted by De Montfort University in England revealed that 93% of infertile men felt depressed, lonely, suicidal, and anxious about a future without children. But nearly 40% of men don't seek support due to social stigma of being macho but incapable of producing children.

Instead of relying on medications all the time for sex or steroids, men can prevent erectile dysfunction and infertility by quitting smoking, eliminating steroids, exercising, eating healthy, avoiding alcohol, reducing stress, and quitting drugs. JustHuynh Fitness' program of martial arts and power athletics can help men stay fit for an enjoyable sex life.

WOMEN SEXUAL DESIRE DISORDER

According to the Cleveland Clinic, 43% of women report sexual dysfunction - having problems with sexual response, desire, orgasm, or pain. Low libido (drive for sexual activity) can result from diabetes, low blood pressure, depression, unhappy relationships, and antidepressants. Hormonally, lower estrogen levels after menopause (when most women's menstrual periods stop and they can no longer bear children - around age 51) lead to decreased blood flow to the pelvic region that leads to less genital sensation.

Per the International Society for Sexual Medicine, 1 in 10 women have HSDD (hypoactive sexual desire disorder) which means low sex drive. Health expert Jennifer Wider says that entrepreneurs are currently working to discover the female equivalent for "Male ED" where drugs target a women's neurotransmitters and chemicals in the brain to increase sexual desire. The potential side effects of existing drugs are nausea, dizziness, fatigue, drop in blood pressure, and fainting when consumed with alcohol.

Cindy Eckert, CEO of Sprout Pharmaceuticals, was inspired to create the first "female viagra" from speaking with hundreds of women suffering from low to non-existent sex drives. Cindy says "I learnt that a lot of these women are in healthy, loving relationships: there's just this one piece that's not working, and that's starting to tear away at the rest of it. Because when things break down in the bedroom, they're often also breaking down at the breakfast table and in other profound ways...reading "Fifty Shades Of Grey" and "buying sexy lingerie" won't solve low libido." However, there is currently no "female viagra" pill that guarantees increase in sexual drive for women.

Women can increase their dopamine by hugging your love partner more, getting sufficient sleep, losing weight, stressing less, and exercising.

SELF LOVE - MASTURBATION

People love to pleasure themselves such as women investing in skin care, manicures, pedicures, plastic surgery, sex toys, and much more whereas men invest in shaving products, golf, hair loss products, erectile dysfunction assistance, wealth management self-help, and much more.

Self love known as achieving orgasm thru masturbation is totally safe and harmless. In fact, some people believe that masturbation should become a regular part of your personal care routine, kind of like brushing your teeth per Gloria Brame - a clinical sexologist. In tandem with exercising, masturbation helps with stress, mood, and maintaining healthy reproductive organs.

Women - if you watched the "Shape of Water" movie, Elisa begins each morning by masturbating in her bathtub. In the film series "Fifty Shades of Grey," Ana enjoys being sexually stimulated by her lover Christian Grey. Scientifically, masturbation eases menopause to prevent narrowing of the vagina, boost blood flow, and relieve tissue problems allowing for better sex.

Men - if you watched the "Wolf of Wall Street" movie, Matthew McConaughey advises his protege Leonardo DiCaprio that the key to success is by "jerking off" or masturbating two times a day. Once in the morning after your workout and another right after lunch to keep your "rhythm flowing." Researchers from the Harvard Chan School of Public Health found that men in their 20s who ejaculated at least 21 times a month were 19 percent less likely to develop prostate cancer and men in their 40s were 22 percent less likely to develop prostate cancer. Masturbation works out your pelvic floor muscles which help prevent erectile dysfunction and incontinence so you don't have to rely on drugs for sexual enhancement. For men who still want to have children, masturbating improves sperm quality as your batches of fresh sperm have less DNA damage and sperm motility problems moving thru the female reproductive tract.

When men or women masturbate, released endorphins help relieve your stresses. Also released are feel-good neurochemicals like dopamine and oxytocin that lift your mood. For relationships, masturbation will heighten your sexual awareness so you can direct your sex partners to stimulate you in the most sensational spots.

RAUNCHY SEX & REVENGE BODY EXERCISES

It's no secret that remaining sexually active has been linked to life satisfaction and longer life. A study published in the British Medical Journal in 1997 found that those with a higher frequency of orgasm had a 50% reduced risk of mortality. Humans need love just like bonobos apes who Primatologist Frans de Waal calls the "make love, not war" species since they resolve most conflicts through sex; and the queen bee who has sex with 200 male drone bees mid-air to build her colony. Being lonely and single can be devastating as lonely people are susceptible to rely on drugs and alcohol to fill the time void that could eventually lead to death.

Many of us get inspired about sex thru magazines such as the Cosmopolitan, Redbook, or Men's Health that cover wild stories such as the Summer Olympics ordering 100,000 condoms for the 10,000 athletes as United States women's soccer goalkeeper Hope Solo and swimmer Ryan Lochte say 75% of Olympians have sex in Olympic Village. Outside of the Olympics, many celebrities go public with their sex life such as New York Yankees Big 5 (Babe Ruth, Mickey Mantle, Reggie Jackson, A-Rod, Derek Jeter) seen with celebrity girlfriends; porn star cougar Lisa Ann revealed in a GQ interview that at age 42 she's had sex with hundreds of freshly drafted 18 to 20-year old NBA players where her rule is to never date more than one guy on a team to avoid locker room gossip and she watches the NBA draft every year to pick out her next sexual conquests - normally targeting the top 3 picks; actor Charlie Sheen who is famous for having sex with over 700 women but unfortunately became the face of HIV when he tested HIV positive from having unprotected sex with one of two women he says, singer Lindsay Lohan having sex with 36 men, Los Angeles Laker legend Magic Johnson admitting in Jerry West's book "West by West" that he had sex with 500 women each year before his HIV diagnosis where he would take women back to the sauna after games to have sex with before doing interviews with the press; singer Taylor Swift told a HollyWood Source that she had amazing sex with former boyfriend Calvin Harris because "He's like the best parts of her exes all wrapped into one. He has the sexual chemistry of John Mayer, the charm of Harry Styles, the heart of Jake Gyllenhaal, and the body of Taylor Lautner;" singer John Mayer told Cazzie David that he's had sex with less than 500 women including Jennifer Aniston, Katy Perry, Jessica Simpson, Jennifer Love Hewitt, and Taylor Swift; singer Madonna said she had amazing sex with Guy Ritchie while paying attention to their BlackBerrys for business, billionaire investor Warren Buffett having "two" wives at once, rapper Nicki Minaj demanding her love partner must be able to have sex with her three times per night, basketball players Wilt Chamberlain citing he had sex with 20,000 women, comedian Amy Schumer being vocal about having sex with 28 men before her marriage, French President Emmanuel Macron marrying his former high school teacher who's 25 years older than him, celebrity Kim Kardashian who made billions for her family from her viral sex video with singer Ray J, Quarterback Tom Brady hinting his sexual antics with Gisele by replying "yes" to Barstool Sports Instagram post of a hippo's mouth kissing his partner's butt, singer Beyonce saying she's "Sasha Fierce in Bed" with Jay Z, model Chrissy Teigen revealing to Cosmopolitan magazine that she and her John Legend joined the "mile high club" for having sex flying first-class, Jada Pinkett Smith telling Redbook that she keeps her marriage strong with Will Smith by having sex in random places like at a girlfriend's house, and both actors Brad Pitt & Angelina Jolie vowing a year of celibacy after divorcing because it would be hard to find another great sex partner.

Khloe Kardashian, who stars in her show "Revenge Body," started the trend of transforming from "fat to fit" after a breakup such as she experienced with Lamar Odom. The show's biggest advice for long-lasting weight-loss is to "attend group fitness classes for the community, teacher, and effective cardio style that you like." Thru exercise, you'll be a "new you" ready to find new love. Other celebrities who've looked "better after breakup" thru exercise are Katie Holmes, Britney Spears, Kourtney Kardashian, Jennifer Garner, Kaley Cuoco, Sofia Vergara, Ciara, Selena Gomez, Jennifer Lawrence, Demi Moore, Heidi Klum, Miranda Lambert, Blac Chyna, Kate Gosselin, Christie Brinkley, Elizabeth Hurley, Eva Longoria, Jordin Sparks, and Halle Berry.

For long-lasting enjoyable sex, some people get creative such as singer Macklemore who has a naked picture of Justin Bieber above his bed to stare at when he's having sex with his wife. Macklemore says "It goes right above my bed and whenever I'm with my wife intimately, I can always stare at it if I want to control my orgasm, just slow it down." Rapper Nicki Minaj stresses the importance of a healthy sex life with her best friends thru sex interventions as Nicki believes every women should reach a climax during sex. Nicki says, "I have a friend who's never had an orgasm in her life. In her life! That hurts my heart. It's cuckoo to me. We always have orgasm interventions where we show her how to do stuff. We'll straddle each other saying 'You gotta get on him like that and do it like this.'"

Sex expert Jennifer Berman who has appeared on comedian Conan O'Brien's show advises men and women on exercises to help top or bottom positions during sex. When on top during missionary position, the plank ab hold and pushups are great exercises to master. When on bottom, the barbell hip thrust and reverse crunches help. For endurance throughout sex, performing martial arts and power athletics thru JustHuynh Fitness' classes is the key to success.

SEX HEALTH BENEFITS

Now with a fit body thru JustHuynh Fitness' martial arts and power athletics, you can enhance your health thru safe sex with love partners.

Lower Stress: Research from the University of the West of Scotland's psychology professor Stuart Brody cite that people who have sex at least once every two weeks manage stressful situations such as public speaking well. Laura Berman, author of "It's Not Him, It's You!," says endorphins and oxytocin released during sex activate pleasure centers in the brain that reduce anxiety and depression.

Relaxation: during sex, the body releases the hormone prolactin that helps with drowsiness for sound sleep.

Pain relief: A study conducted at the Headache Clinic at Southern Illinois University found that half of female migraine sufferers reported relief after climaxing due to the released endorphins resembling morphine. In a study by Rutgers sex researcher Beverly Whipple, who coined the term "G-spot," studies found that the pressure of pleasurable vaginal stimulation increased pain tolerance by 40% and increased by 75% when the women reached orgasm.

Fewer illnesses: According to researchers at Wilkes University, people who have sex have higher levels of an antibody called "immunoglobulin A" that help keep the body safe from colds and the flu.

Healthy heart: According to a study by the New England Research Institute, men who have sex at least two times a week are 45% less likely to have heart disease than men who have sex only once a month or less. For women, Hui Liu of Michigan State University found that sex protects older women from cardiovascular risk later in life and also lower risk of hypertension (high blood pressure).

Smarts: British researchers, from the English Longitudinal Study of Ageing, found that men and women between the ages 50 and 89 who have sex at least once a week, had increased cognitive function when measured by number sequencing and word recall.

Beautiful face: sexologist Dr. Gloria G. Bramer says an orgasm a day pumps oxygen to your skin for rosier cheeks and produces collagen that keeps your face wrinkle free.

Young look: Dr. Yvonne Fulbright, author of "The Better Sex Guide to Extraordinary Love Making," cites a 10 year study on 3,500 men and women that revealed those with an active sex life had their age underestimated by seven to 12 years, while the group that had sex infrequently looked older.

Longer telomeres: telomeres are DNA strand protectors. A person with short telomeres are susceptible to developing a degenerative disease or die young. Tomás Cabeza de Baca of the University of California, San Francisco cites a study that looked at 129 mothers in committed relationships over the course of a week to assess overall relationship satisfaction, stress, partner support, and intimacy. In the study, women who had sex once a week had significantly longer telomeres. This held true even when adjusting for other factors such as perceived stress and relationship quality.

Success: In Napoleon Hill's book "Think and Grow Rich," Napoleon says "Sex desire is the most powerful of human desires. When driven by this desire, men develop keenness of imagination, courage, will-power, persistence, and creative ability unknown to them at other times."

CHAPTER 23

LUCID DREAMS

All men dream, but not equally. Those who dream by night in the dusty recesses of their minds, wake in the day to find that it was vanity: but the dreamers of the day are dangerous men, for they may act on their dreams with open eyes, to make them possible

- T.E. Lawrence

SLEEP SATISFACTION

With 24 hours in a day, it is recommended that you get at least six hours of sleep a night for proper recovery. Spending about a third of our lives asleep and considering the average United States-born person lives until age 80, that means you spend about 26 years of your life asleep.

What if you could have total control of your dreams? That is what's called having a lucid dream where you are the director and star of your own movie in your dreams. Lucid dreams allow you to be actively exploring, learning, and growing while you're asleep making the most of your time. This is a technique that has been practiced by Buddhists for thousands of years where regular exercise helps you sleep deeper and dream better during REM.

When sleeping, you want your body temperature leveled and your adrenaline low so that it's easier for you to wind down. So if you're a person who exercises at night, your heart rate and body temperature will be high. You can lower your body temperature by taking a long, cool shower post-workout to help you with lucid dreams.

ACHIEVE ANYTHING

Research shows that in a lucid dream your brain thinks you're actually doing what you're dreaming which has helped people lose weight, treat stress, confront phobias, and achieve career goals such as turning from employee to entrepreneur. Lucid dreams are even more powerful than athletes who use visualization training to improve their performance.

Research shows that memory works best when something is learned shortly before sleep. Fill your brain with new ideas and inspiration; related to your love life, academics, athletics, or business; before bed such as from reading a book that will give your mind work to do while you're asleep.

Personally, I read success stories from business folks I admire before bed and always look at my motivational wall that has Sam Walton, Steve Jobs, Bruce Lee, and Super saiyan Goku to achieve my goal of helping the world get healthy thru JustHuynh Fitness' martial arts and power athletics. If you're looking to boost confidence, gain self defense skills, stay healthy, improve intellectually, thrive professionally, strengthen your love life, and age gracefully, JustHuynh Fitness would love to help you achieve your life goals.

ABOUT THE AUTHOR

Francis Huynh is CEO & Founder of JustHuynh - a social fitness company that helps people just win at health by training together for the needed social accountability and motivation in achieving their fitness goals thru martial arts and power athletics. JustHuynh provides in-home/online personal training and onsite/studio group fitness to help clients reduce risks of obesity, ageing, and mental health. Obesity is personal - as Francis went thru childhood obesity at Age 10, the college freshman 15 (the phenomenon where students gain 15 pounds during first year in college) at Age 18, and Working Adult Obesity (couch potato laziness) at Age 22. His life changed when his doctor diagnosed him as obese. From that moment, Francis started prioritizing exercise and nutrition - realizing that fitness provides benefits of benefits that allow anyone to thrive instead of just surviving at life.

In 2016 after marrying the love of his life and completing MBA degree from the fittest/brightest university in the world (Vanderbilt), Francis turned down lucrative career opportunities (i.e. FBI, Samsung) to pursue his passion and calling of empowering people to escape the treadmill of mediocrity onto the fast track to success by improving their nutrition and exercise with JustHuynh Fitness.

If you want to lose weight, reverse ageing, get strong, and improve mental health, Francis and his team are committed to helping you achieve your health goals with martial arts, power athletics, and healthy life habits.

Outside of work, Francis enjoys spending time with family, paying it forward thru community service (i.e. helping people with fitness, education, cultural awareness, business, overcoming challenges as a 1st Generation college graduate), practicing martial arts, traveling globally, and reading business books.

www.francishuynh.com

AUTHOR'S NOTES

In many ways, this book began thirty years ago when I was born in Maine United States to parents who came over as boat people after surviving as South Vietnamese prisoners of war during the Vietnam War.

My journey as a 1st generation Asian American to make my parents proud, who saved their entire earnings from low-wage blue collar jobs for my brother and I to achieve the "American Dream" thru education and merit, was made uneasy from racism and discrimination.

This book is based on history and my personal experiences to help anyone improve their life personally and professionally by boosting confidence, intellect, youthfulness, and self-defense skills thru JustHuynh Fitness' martial arts and power athletics where you'll transform into an "Ageless Athletic Assassin."

I am also grateful to authors of outstanding books, articles, movies, speeches, studies, and news stories - and have honored each author in the text of this book.

SERVICES FROM JUSTHUYNH FITNESS

Speaking Event
Minimum audience of 250 people for 45-minute workout and 30-minute Q&A. Ideal for conferences, companies, colleges, concerts, community
LINK → www.francishuynh.com/fitnesstour

Online Training Program (Monthly Membership)
Receive 3 strength and 3 cardio workouts each week to achieve an "Ageless Athletic Assassin" fitness level that can be performed in your home gym
LINK → www.francishuynh.com/444to200

Fitness Studio (Monthly Membership)
JustHuynh Fitness monthly membership providing 12 classes a month of martial arts and power athletics. Gift Certificates also available for friends.
LINK → www.justhuynh.com

Licensee Studio Opportunity
Open a licensed JustHuynh Fitness studio in your city to teach our signature martial arts and power athletics program
LINK → www.justhuynh.com/become-a-licensee

In-Home Gym Equipment List
You can perform all workouts at home. All you need is treadmill (min 12 mph/20 km), bench press set, dumbbells, kickboxing bag, and boxing gloves
LINK → www.francishuynh.com/vlogblog/best-home-gym-equipment-2018

Workout Gear
Rock JustHuynh Fitness gear: t-shirt, sweater, and more.
LINK → www.francishuynh.com/gear

Social Media
Instagram → franciskhuynh
Weibo → franciskhuynh
Newsletter (Products, etc.) → www.francishuynh.com/newslettersignup

www.ingramcontent.com/pod-product-compliance
Lightning Source LLC
Chambersburg PA
CBHW060315030426
42336CB00011B/1059